THE EUROPEAN PATIENT
OF THE FUTURE

STATE OF HEALTH SERIES

Edited by Chris Ham, Professor of Health Policy and Management at the University of Birmingham and Director of the Strategy Unit at the Department of Health.

Current and forthcoming titles

THE EUROPEAN PATIENT OF THE FUTURE

EDITED BY
Angela Coulter and Helen Magee

Open University Press
Maidenhead · Philadelphia

Open University Press
McGraw-Hill Education
McGraw-Hill House
Shoppenhangers Road
Maidenhead
Berkshire
England
SL6 2QL

email: enquiries@openup.co.uk
world wide web: www.openup.co.uk

and
325 Chestnut Street
Philadelphia, PA 19106, USA

First Published 2003

A catalogue record of this book is available from the British Library

ISBN 0 335 21187 9 (pb)   0 335 21188 7 (hb)

Library of Congress Cataloging-in-Publication Data
CIP data has been applied for

Typeset by RefineCatch Limited, Bungay, Suffolk
Printed in Great Britain by Bell & Bain Ltd, Glasgow

CONTENTS

RESEARCHERS AND OTHER CONTRIBUTORS

GERMANY

Researchers

Marie-Luise Dierks, Dept of Epidemiology, Social Medicine and Health System Research, Hanover Medical School
Gabriele Schwarz, Dept of Epidemiology, Social Medicine and Health System Research, Hanover Medical School

Advisers

Dr Holland, Ministry of Health
Dr Erwin Dehlinger, Federal Association of Sickness Funds, Berlin
Dr Justine Engelbrecht, Chamber of Physicians
Henriette Hentschel, Merck Sharp and Dohme Germany
Dr Günther Holling, patient counsellor
Dr Erwin Nachtigäller, Cooperation of Disabled People, Cologne
Dr Thomas Ruprecht, Picker Institute Germany
Professor Friedrich-Wilhelm Schwartz, Hanover Medical School
Frau Karin Stötzner, Coordinating Centre for Self-Help Groups, Berlin

ITALY

Researchers

Roberta Barletta, Fondazione Centro Studi Investimenti Sociali (CENSIS)

Carla Collicelli, Fondazione Centro Studi Investimenti Sociali (CENSIS)
Maria Concetta Vaccaro, Fondazione Centro Studi Investimenti Sociali (CENSIS)

Advisers

Dr Simona Alunni, Merck Sharp and Dohme Italy
Dr Ivan Cavicchi, Farmindustria
Dr Mario Falconi, Italian Federation of General Medicine
Dr Stefano Inglese, Tribunal for Patients' Rights
Prof. Sandro Spinsanti, L'Arco di Giano

POLAND

Researchers

Alexandra Banaszewska, National Centre for Quality Assessment in Healthcare, Cracow
Jacek Siwiec, National Centre for Quality Assessment in Healthcare, Cracow

Contributors

Piotr Cieślik, National Centre for Quality Assessment in Healthcare, Cracow
Jacek Walczak, National Centre for Quality Assessment in Healthcare, Cracow

Advisers

Elżbieta Bobiatyńska, National Centre for Health Information Systems, Warsaw
Janusz Halik, National Centre for Health Information Systems, Warsaw
Rafał Niżankowski, Polish Society for Quality Promotion in Healthcare in Poland, Cracow
Andrzej Pajak, Institute of Public Health, Cracow
Jolanta Sabbat, Merck Sharp and Dohme Poland

SLOVENIA

Researchers

Dr Tit Albreht, Institute of Public Health of the Republic of Slovenia
Janja Sesok, Institute of Public Health of the Republic of Slovenia
Jana Trdic, Institute of Public Health of the Republic of Slovenia
Nevenka Kelsin, Institute of Public Health of the Republic of Slovenia

Contributor

Mojca Gruntar Cinc, Ministry of Health

Advisers

Tjasa Burnik, Merck Sharp and Dohme Slovenia
Andreja Cufar, Slovenian Pharmaceutical Society
Bojana Filej, Nursing Chamber of Slovenia
Boris Kramberger, Health Insurance Institute of Slovenia
Breda Kutin, Consumer Association of Slovenia
Dr Dorjan Marusic, Ministry of Health
Dr Andrej Mozina, Medical Chamber of Slovenia
Dr Janez Remskar, Association of Public Providers of Healthcare
Diana Zajec, Delo

SPAIN

Researcher

Albert Jovell, Josep Laporte Foundation

Contributors

Angeles Barrios, Merck Sharp and Dohme Spain
Mireia Molina, Técnicas de Grupo, Madrid
Eduardo Montesinos, Técnicas de Grupo, Madrid
Antoni Gelonch, Merck Sharp and Dohme Spain
Francesc Roig, Josep Laporte Foundation

SWEDEN

Researchers

Lars Fallberg, Picker Institute Scandinavia
Per Rosén, Skane Region

Advisers

Marie-Jeanette Bergvall, Infomedica
Peter Garpenby, University of Linköping
Marianne Lidbrink, Swedish Nurses Association
Johan Thor, Karolinska Institute

SWITZERLAND

Researchers

Jen Wang, Institute for Social and Preventative Medicine, Zurich University
Federico Cathieni, Institute for Social and Preventative Medicine, Lausanne University
Laurence Peer, Institute for Social and Preventative Medicine, Lausanne University
M. Béatrice Cordonier, Institute for Social and Preventative Medicine, Lausanne University
Karin Werner, Institute for Social and Preventative Medicine, Zurich University
Valérie Hiniker, Institute for Social and Preventative Medicine, Lausanne University
Bernard Burnand Institute for Social and Preventative Medicine, Lausanne University

Advisers

Sergio Belluci, Swiss Science and Technology Council
Hans-Heinrich Brunner, Swiss Medical Association
Gianfranco Domenighetti, Ticino Health Department
Reto Guetg, Association of Swiss Sickness Funds
Yvonne Husemann, Picker Institute Switzerland
Gerhard Kocher, Swiss Society for Health Policy
Manfred Langenegger, Swiss Federal Office of Social Insurance

Marianne Meyer, Consumers Association (Romandie)
Catherine Panchaud, Swiss Nursing Association
Dominique Sprumont, Universities of Neuchâtel and Fribourg
K. Rodegra, Merck Sharp and Dohme Switzerland
Stefan Wild, Merck Sharp and Dohme Switzerland
Thomas Zeltner, Swiss Federal Office of Public Health
Erwin Zimmerman, University of Neuchâtel

UNITED KINGDOM

Researchers

Liz Kendall, Institute for Public Policy Research
Laura Edwards, Institute for Public Policy Research

Contributor

Jo Lenaghan, Institute for Public Policy Research

Advisers

Prof. Angela Coulter, Picker Institute Europe
Anne Damerell, Pain Concern
Dr Simon Fradd, British Medical Association
Bob Gann, NHS Direct Online
Pippa Gough, King's Fund
Angela Hayes, International Alliance of Patients' Organizations
Susan Lewis, Gauchers Association
Clara McKay, Consumers' Association
Sir Alexander Macara, National Heart Forum and University of
    York
Gopa Mitra, Proprietary Association of Great Britain
Barrie Taylor, Community Health Councils Development Association
Matthew Taylor, Institute for Public Policy Research
Kate Tillett, Merck Sharp & Dohme UK

The study was funded by an unrestricted educational grant from
Merck & Co., Inc., New Jersey, USA, which is known outside North
America as Merck Sharp & Dohme (MSD). We are grateful to them
for making it possible, and in particular to Jeffrey L. Sturchio and
Melinda Hanisch for coordinating the contribution from the MSD

local offices and for advice and support throughout the project. Grateful thanks are also due to Prof. Alan Williams for help in recruiting researchers, to Remco Frerichs and Wiene Klasema of NIPO for organizing the telephone survey, and to Prof. Crispin Jenkinson for help with analysing the survey data.

SERIES EDITOR'S INTRODUCTION

Health services in many developed countries have come under critical scrutiny in recent years. In part this is because of increasing expenditure, much of it funded from public sources, and the pressure this has put on governments seeking to control public spending. Also important has been the perception that resources allocated to health services are not always deployed in an optimal fashion. Thus at a time when the scope for increasing expenditure is extremely limited, there is a need to search for ways of using existing budgets more efficiently. A further concern has been the desire to ensure access to health care of various groups on an equitable basis. In some countries this has been linked to a wish to enhance patient choice and to make service providers more responsive to patients as 'consumers'.

Underlying these specific concerns are a number of more fundamental developments which have a significant bearing on the performance of health services. Three are worth highlighting. First, there are demographic changes, including the ageing population and the decline in the proportion of the population of working age. These changes will both increase the demand for health care and at the same time limit the ability of health services to respond to this demand.

Second, advances in medical science will also give rise to new demands within the health services. These advances cover a range of possibilities, including innovations in surgery, drug therapy, screening and diagnosis. The pace of innovation is likely to quicken, with significant implications for the funding and provision of services.

Third, public expectations of health services are rising as those who use services demand higher standards of care. In part, this is stimulated by developments within the health service, including the availability of new technology. More fundamentally, it stems from the emergence of a more educated and informed population, in which people are accustomed to being treated as consumers rather than patients.

Against this background, policy makers in a number of countries are reviewing the future of health services. Those countries which have traditionally relied on a market in health care are making greater use of regulation and planning. Equally, those countries which have traditionally relied on regulation and planning are moving towards a more competitive approach. In no country is there complete satisfaction with existing methods of financing and delivery, and everywhere there is a search for new policy instruments.

The aim of this series is to contribute to debate about the future of health services through an analysis of major issues in health policy. These issues have been chosen because they are both of current interest and of enduring importance. The series is intended to be accessible to students and informed lay readers as well as to specialists working in this field. The aim is to go beyond a textbook approach to health policy analysis and to encourage authors to move debate about their issue forward. In this sense, each book presents a summary of current research and thinking, and an exploration of future policy directions.

Professor Chris Ham
Professor of Health Policy and Management
University of Birmingham

1

INTRODUCTION

PUBLIC RESPONSE TO FUTURE TRENDS

We are living through a period of profound change in the way in which health services are organized, delivered and experienced. Developments in biotechnology have led to many new and more effective treatments. Genetic research holds out the hope of even better ways of diagnosing and treating disease. New applications of information technology offer opportunities to extend and speed up the delivery of health care.

These technological advances are affecting, and are affected by, wider sociocultural changes. People are better informed, less deferential to professionals and those in authority and more willing to complain if services aren't up to scratch. Consumerism is apparent in many areas of public life and health care is no exception. Health services in all European countries are now experiencing an unprecedented level of demand, partly due to demographic change and partly the result of greater awareness of what might be on offer.

It is often said that public expectations are rising, but what exactly does this mean? Medical care has never been so abundant or so effective, yet dissatisfaction and complaints appear to be increasing. What do patients want and how feasible will it be to meet their demands? In their efforts to reform health systems, politicians are hoping to narrow the gap between public expectations and the capacity of the system to deliver. What must they do to make health services more responsive and more effective, yet affordable?

This book describes a study carried out in eight European countries (Germany, Italy, Poland, Slovenia, Spain, Sweden,

Switzerland and the UK) that set out to find answers to these questions. We wanted to learn more about the concerns of European patients: what they liked and disliked about the health systems in their countries, what roles they wanted to play in their own care and in shaping health policy, and how they would react to changes that are likely to take place in the near future which will affect the way they experience health care.

Policy dilemmas

Priorities differ in different European countries, but policy makers are grappling with many of the same issues. Our study aimed to look at common policy dilemmas through the eyes of the patient. We wanted to know what patients and the public perceived to be the most pressing problems, and to explore their reactions to specific approaches to tackling them. How confident did they feel about the capacity of health systems to deliver the amount and quality of health care that they believe they will need? Could they pinpoint specific deficiencies in the systems and would they be willing to pay more to put them right? To what extent would people tolerate increased taxes or higher insurance premiums to pay for more or better health care? How acceptable are current levels of out-of-pocket payments and would people be willing to contemplate paying directly for an increased range of services?

If health systems are to adapt to the new demands, people will be required to make trade-offs between different values. We wanted to find out what kind of trade-offs people might be willing to make. For example, would they be willing to trade continuity of care from a known and trusted source (e.g. their family doctor) for faster access from a wider range of providers? How would patients respond to changes in staff skill mix or extensions of professional roles? Does the desire for greater involvement in decision making mean that people are willing to take on more responsibility for their own health care, and, if so, how can self-care be supported? How can patients' information needs be met and will the internet make things easier or more difficult? Information technology offers the potential to store vast amounts of data and access it quickly, but what about the desire for privacy and confidentiality: can this be safeguarded? How important is individual choice and how do people weigh that up against equity of access? How will new technologies such as genetic screening impact on future demand for services, and how acceptable will they be? New treatment technologies hold out the hope of more effective ways of dealing with illness, but does this mean that time for personal communication and empathy must inevitably become more restricted? What reactions can be expected to the various attempts to manage demand – for example, by introducing gatekeeping systems or rationing access to certain treatments or services? And to what extent do members of the public want to get engaged in policy debates and in finding solutions to these problems?

These questions are relevant in most western countries, but the responses to them may differ between countries. For example, patients' views and behaviour may be influenced by the type of health system and the way it is funded (i.e. by taxation, social insurance or private insurance). The relationship between patients and clinicians may be influenced by the extent to which patients are currently expected to pay out-of-pocket costs – for example, for GP consultations or for prescribed drugs, or by the extent of competition between providers. Other health policy differences may also impact on patients' expectations – for example, the extent to which patients' rights are promoted and publicized, or the relative amount of freedom patients have to choose who to consult about health problems (e.g. free access to specialists versus a gatekeeping system). Technology diffusion is occurring at different paces in different countries. New medicines come onto the market more quickly in some countries than in others and the use of information technology is more advanced in some places than in others. More fundamentally, the extent to which patient empowerment and public engagement with policy making is on the policy agenda varies considerably between European countries, which could be both a cause and a consequence of differences in attitudes and expectations.

Our aims in undertaking the international comparisons were threefold. First, we wanted to develop a better understanding of the future role of patients in particular countries, and the potential impact that these developments may have on future health care policy within the respective countries. Second, we hoped to identify differences between patients' expectations and preferences so as to understand better the drivers and obstacles to change. Finally, we hoped that by extending our research beyond the confines of one country or one type of patient, we would avoid simplistic conclusions that were not applicable elsewhere.

FUTURE SCENARIOS

Attempting to forecast health trends is a difficult and risky business. Extrapolating future developments in patients' expectations from incomplete knowledge of their current concerns can lead policy makers down blind alleys. One only has to remember the mistakes of the recent past to see the pitfalls. For example, in the UK a belief that patients preferred to be treated at home, or as near to home as possible, was used to justify reductions in hospital bed numbers which proved highly unpopular and is now having to be rectified.[1] And the assumption that patients (and their GPs) would be willing to shop around to find the best quality care led to disillusion with GP fundholding when public concerns about equity proved a more powerful driver.[2]

Nevertheless, this is a minefield through which health policy makers have to tread. All health systems use public funds to a greater or lesser extent and all, therefore, depend on public consensus for their sustainability. The policy debate in European countries has centred on various ways of adapting the systems to deal with scarcity of resources while ensuring the continuation of public support. Examples include cost-sharing arrangements, rationing access to certain services, incentives for private spending, and other ways of reducing demand by shifting costs onto the individual.[3] Many countries have made changes to their funding systems, some of which have been quite fundamental.[4] Other reform strategies have included the introduction of competition among health care providers, setting global expenditure ceilings, controlling numbers of staff or beds, controlling the cost of pharmaceuticals, employing cheaper staff, substituting outpatient and primary care for more expensive inpatient services, regulating the use of technologies or changing the way professionals are remunerated.

All these initiatives impact on patients and the public in one way or another. Our study looked for evidence on how health service users might respond to various scenarios, some of which they might have experienced themselves, while others were more hypothetical. These included the possibility that patients might be required to pay more direct out-of-pocket payments for various health care services, that nurses and pharmacists might take over roles which were previously the exclusive province of doctors, that new services such as complementary therapies and genetic screening might be either incorporated into (or excluded from) the current package, that patients would be encouraged to play a greater role in their own care and in choosing treatments, that they would want to be able to choose their health care providers, and that citizens might be expected to have a view about rights and responsibilities and to participate in debates about how to ration health care. These scenarios are considered in more detail below.

Willingness to pay more

Expenditure on health care has been rising fast in most European countries,[5] but public concerns about quality and access do not always coincide with willingness to increase contributions to enable these problems to be tackled, even when people believe that underfunding is the root cause.[6] Where taxation provides the main source of funding people tend not to vote for political parties that promise to increase income tax. In countries where the health system is based on social insurance, neither employers nor employees are keen to contemplate increases in the burden of insurance contributions.

The arguments against increasing co-payments or encouraging 'top-up' insurance as a means of narrowing the gap between demand and supply usually centre on concerns about equity.[7] We were interested to know whether this concern was still predominant in the minds of European patients, or whether increasing affluence has resulted in a greater willingness to contribute out-of-pocket payments. Are people still firmly attached to the solidarity principle that characterizes European health systems? How much public support is there for market-based systems and more competition in health care? Would people tolerate greater inequalities in access to care in return for the freedom (for those who could afford it) to buy an extended range of services, to obtain faster access, or to opt out of public health care altogether?

New professional roles

The roles of doctors, nurses and pharmacists have been changing over recent years in response to technological developments and changes in the way health care is organized. Communications technology has enabled better, faster record keeping and medical notes can now be accessed from different locations and by different groups of clinical staff. Access to research evidence and treatment protocols is now far easier, and improvements in education systems have enhanced people's ability to adapt to these new developments. As health care becomes more complex and more expensive, specialization has increased and the need for different groups of professional staff to coordinate their activities has become more urgent. Professional roles have been reassessed in the search for a more effective and efficient division of labour.[8] The changes have been further stimulated by pressure from these groups of staff as they manoeuvre to maintain and strengthen their position.

The family doctor is still ubiquitous and highly regarded, but the traditional single-handed practitioner is fast disappearing in many European countries, to be replaced by group practices located in health centres. These often employ a wide range of primary care professionals and others with specialist skills, with access to increasingly sophisticated diagnostic and therapeutic equipment. General practice as a medical specialty exists everywhere in Europe but its nature and position in the medical hierarchy differs from country to country. In countries where GPs have achieved a relatively powerful position, their strength rests on the loyalty of their patients underpinned by their gatekeeping function – the referral system in which patients cannot consult a specialist without a letter from a GP – that protects them against competition from hospital-based specialists. Many European governments are trying to introduce gatekeeping or managed care systems where these previously did not exist because a strong primary care system is seen as conveying efficiency benefits.[9] However, these sit uneasily alongside countervailing pressures to encourage freedom of choice for patients, including the freedom to consult any doctor.

Nowadays, nurse training is more academic than it used to be. Nurses no longer want to be seen merely as doctors' assistants. Instead they see themselves as well qualified professionals working alongside doctors in a complementary rather than subordinate role. Many feel confident to take on extended responsibilities. For example, nurse practitioners in primary care may take sole responsibility for the care of certain patients, triage schemes give nurses responsibility for making initial diagnoses in many settings, some nurses are being given the right to prescribe certain treatments and there are now specialist nurses in many fields who provide the main source of information and support for patients with life-threatening diseases such as cancer, heart disease or stroke.

Changes in the pharmacist's role have been driven by developments in the way medicines are packaged and distributed. They no longer have to make up medicinal compounds or count out individual pills because most drugs arrive pre-packaged. Highly trained in chemistry and pharmacy, they are often more knowledge-able than doctors about how drugs work and the side-effects and contra-indications. Many have become shopkeepers, selling a wide range of products in addition to prescribed or over-the-counter medicines, but some feel their skills are underutilized. They and their professional bodies have been pushing for a wider role in medicine monitoring, prescribing, health advice and prevention.

We were keen to find out what patients thought about these new developments. Would they be happy to consult nurses instead of doctors for some problems? Should pharmacists be allowed to prescribe medicines? How important is continuity of care? Would patients be willing to trade-off the one-to-one relationship with their family doctor against the possibility of faster access to any one of a group of doctors?

Remote access to health advice

The telephone is not a new technology, but the establishment of telephone helplines to provide an alternative access route to medical advice is a relatively new development. For example, in some countries there are helplines staffed by health professionals who are available 24-hours a day to enable patients to seek advice about any aspect of their health care.[10] People can phone with queries on a wide range of issues. Callers can describe symptoms they are experiencing and ask for advice on what's wrong with them, parents may phone for suggestions on how to deal with a crying baby, others may want a second opinion on treatment advice they have received, or informa-tion on the side-effects of medicines they have been prescribed, or help in locating specific services. Structured computer protocols are often used to help the advisers answer the wide range of queries received and to ensure that those with urgent needs are directed to the appropriate emergency service.

We wanted to explore patients' views of these helplines together with other ways of accessing health advice remotely – for example, consultations via email, video phones or telemedicine. Great claims have been made for telemedicine, which is said to offer the potential to make the best use of highly skilled expertise to enhance quality of care and reduce differences in treatment and outcome.[11] The combination of computer and communications technologies looks exciting, but what do patients think? Could these alternative ways of accessing specialist advice provide a more efficient and acceptable means of meeting needs, perhaps leading to a reduction in consultation rates and in waiting times in doctors' clinics?

Regulating tests and treatments

The development of new medicines and biotechnologies will continue to widen the scope of what can be done in medical care in relation to diagnosis and treatment, raising important questions about ethics, priorities and cost-effectiveness. New technologies are being developed and promoted commercially and policy makers have to decide whether or not to concede to pressures to extend the scope of reimbursable medical care to include such things as alternative and complementary therapies, new medicines designed for previously 'untreatable' conditions such as impotence or baldness, or self-diagnosis kits and genetic profiling.

In response to growing popular demand for complementary medicine, governments and health authorities are gradually being persuaded to take account of it in their health plans. Despite the popularity of complementary or alternative medicine, orthodox medical practitioners have long resisted its incorporation into the package of reimbursed therapies. But this resistance is beginning to crumble in the face of public demand. Complementary practitioners operate for the most part outside the traditional health systems, but some traditionally-trained health professionals have studied the complementary therapies and now offer them alongside more orthodox treatments. There have been many calls for a more integrated approach which would combine orthodox and complementary therapies within the same system, providing reimbursement for all types of therapies according to agreed rules.

Paradoxically, this trend towards greater recognition of the role of complementary therapies comes at a time when evidence-based medicine is in the ascendancy and professionals are more aware than ever before of the need for critical evaluation of the effects of medical interventions.[12] There is also growing awareness of the requirement to strengthen regulation procedures for all types of practitioners. Policy makers are increasingly concerned to ensure that patient safety is not compromised and that public money is not wasted on ineffective or harmful treatments. In many cases professional self-regulatory systems are under assault and pressure is growing to introduce stronger systems for external regulation of doctors, nurses and other health professionals.

The popularity of largely unevaluated complementary treatments provided by mostly unregulated practitioners is occurring in the face of these policy trends. Complementary medicine is not free at the point of use and it is often scorned by orthodox practitioners. What is the basis of its popular appeal? Does it reflect public disdain for, or mistrust of, orthodox science or concerns about the way in which traditional medicine is delivered? Or is it indicative of a desire for more autonomy and choice, or for greater opportunities for self-help? What will happen if integration becomes the norm and complementary medicine is brought into the fold of scientific evaluation and regulation? Will it lose its appeal? Our study provided an opportunity to explore these issues by looking at public responses in countries where complementary medicine has been treated with different degrees of toleration or encouragement.

There are differences between countries in the speed at which new treatments or diagnostic technologies are adopted. Like complementary therapies, new medicines and biotechnologies are often greeted with a mixture of enthusiasm and suspicion. We wanted to learn more about people's views of these new developments. Did they feel well-informed about the new technologies and new medicines and did they feel confident that they or their children would benefit from them? The particular case study we explored in detail in this study was genetic screening, on which public opinion is known to be divided.[13] Advances in genetics have made it possible to identify disease susceptibility in currently healthy people and genetic testing is beginning to be made more widely available. Presymptomatic testing offers considerable potential for early intervention and prevention.[14] We asked participants in the focus groups which were organized in each of the eight countries to consider their reactions to the wider availability of genetic screening. How would they react to knowing more about the likelihood of developing a life-threatening disease some time in the future? Would they find this prospect alarming or reassuring? What impact would it have on their behaviour?

Promoting patient autonomy

Public demand for health information is widespread and largely unsatisfied. There is a vast array of patient information materials available, but it is not well distributed and much of it is of poor quality.[15] Governments and health authorities have long recognized the need to make available health education materials as part of their attempts to prevent disease and promote healthy lifestyles.

There is now a growing recognition that provision of information about diseases, treatment options and self-help strategies could also be useful as part of a demand management strategy.[16] The hope is that better informed patients will use health services more efficiently and effectively.

The internet offers the potential to meet the demand for information in new and more flexible ways. Yet, it in turn raises problems of inequitable access and quality assurance. Internet access is becoming more widespread, but distribution is patchy and skewed in favour of younger, wealthier and more educated people. Its global spread makes it very difficult to regulate and it is hard for patients to determine the reliability of information on health websites. The online health care industry is dominated by commercial interests. Companies which are trying to sell products often fail to provide balanced information about risks and side-effects. If left unchecked and unchallenged, current developments in information provision could increase demand for inappropriate medical interventions, causing harm to patients and increasing pressures on scarce health care resources.

There is growing evidence that many patients are no longer willing to remain passive recipients of care.[17] Instead there are demands for greater choice and more involvement in decision making. The demand for over-the-counter medicines and complementary therapies is evidence that many people are unwilling to be solely dependent on medical practitioners when they are ill, preferring self-care and self-medication when possible. We aimed to explore the extent of demand for these self-help strategies and to examine how far patients in the different countries felt empowered to look after themselves and to participate in decisions about their care.

The introduction of competition into health systems requires the encouragement of consumerism if these quasi-market mechanisms are to operate effectively.[18] Patients may be offered a choice of payers – i.e. choosing between different health plans or insurance packages, or a choice of providers – i.e. choosing a hospital, specialist or primary care provider. In future we may see more initiatives designed to encourage patients to 'shop around', making choices on the basis of quality, or speed of access, or cost. Following the Kohl and Dekker rulings, people who live in European Union (EU) countries may also have the right to travel to other EU countries for health care.[19] If this is to occur, the public will have to be provided with information on which to base these choices. We explored these ideas with participants in our focus groups to find out the extent of demand for this type of information and choice.

Maintaining public confidence

All European governments have to ensure that the social consensus, without which collective health care provision would be impossible, remains intact and that policy developments are in tune with wider social values. It is seen as important that citizens and the electorate understand the basis of health care reforms and feel informed about policy changes and their underlying justification.

In several of our study countries there have been recent initiatives to secure greater public involvement in policy debates as policy makers attempt to ensure that any restrictions on the growth and availability of health services strike an acceptable balance in the eyes of the public as legitimate trade-offs between the supply of services and the expenditure of public funds. In most countries there have also been attempts to strengthen patients' rights and to publicize these. Attempts to open up the rationing debate have been few and far between, however.[20] Among our study countries, there have been formal attempts to promote public discussion about rationing or 'priority-setting' in Sweden, and the UK government has expressed its intention to do so by setting up a Citizen's Council, but for the most part politicians have shied away from tackling the issue in a transparent manner.

We looked for examples of successful attempts at engaging the public in policy debates and we wanted to know how far people were aware of their rights and felt able to use existing mechanisms to secure them. Overall, we were interested in the extent to which members of the public in these countries felt confident about the future of their health systems, and the likelihood that their future needs and expectations would be met.

STUDY METHODS

There were three main strands to the project: literature reviews, focus groups and a telephone survey. Lead researchers were recruited in each of the eight countries and they were responsible for carrying out the reviews and commissioning the focus group research. The UK study, which was designed by Jo Lenaghan and led by Liz Kendall of the Institute for Public Policy Research in London, commenced in June 2000, a year earlier than elsewhere, and acted as a pilot for the wider European project, which was coordinated by Angela Coulter and Helen Magee of Picker Institute Europe in Oxford.

Advisory groups

The researchers were asked to recruit a small group of experts in each country to provide advice and feedback during the course of the research (see pp. vi–xi). Advisory group members provided a sounding board for the researchers and a 'reality check' as the findings of the reviews and focus groups emerged and were refined.

Literature reviews

Researchers had the task of identifying published papers or media reports that provided evidence on patient and public views of the health care system in their countries. They were encouraged to look for population surveys and other research studies which could shed light on the questions posed above. Templates were developed to ensure that the literature reviews adopted a similar format in each of the countries (see Appendix a).

The quantity and quality of relevant studies differed between the countries. In some there was a great deal of relevant material and researchers had to be selective, while in others there was very little. The literature reviews, which were each about 10,000 words in length, were translated into English and forwarded to the study coordinators in Oxford.

Focus groups

A topic guide was developed for use in the focus groups (see Appendix b). This included descriptions of various scenarios that were used to gauge participants' reactions to likely future developments. The review templates and topic guide were discussed at a meeting in London attended by all the researchers, and final refinements were agreed before the main work began.

Focus groups included participants who were current patients and those whose experience of using the health care system was less immediate. The study teams were asked to try to recruit a good mix of participants in terms of sex, age and socioeconomic group.

Wherever possible, the groups took place in different parts of the relevant country, but with relatively small numbers of groups in each country it wasn't possible to cover all geographical regions. For example, the UK groups all took place in England with no representation from Scotland, Wales or Northern Ireland. In Switzerland, groups were organized in the French-speaking part of the country as well as in German-speaking areas, but not in the Italian-speaking part.

The group discussions lasted anything from one to three hours. In some groups it wasn't possible to cover all the topics included in the topic guide, while in others certain topics were considered in greater depth than others. The discussions were recorded, transcribed and analysed in the relevant country, and then translated into English and forwarded to the coordinators for incorporation into the country reports.

Stakeholder seminars

Once the reviews were complete, seminars were held in each of the countries to present the results to a wider group of key stakeholders to test out ideas and identify areas of agreement and difference in relation to possible policy developments. The finished reviews and focus group reports were edited down from about 20,000 words describing public views in each country to form the individual chapters that appear in this book.

Telephone survey

To supplement the qualitative data obtained from the focus groups and to facilitate the international comparisons, we commissioned a telephone survey of a random sample of the population in each of the countries. Telephone interviews have to be relatively short – ideally they should last no longer than 15 to 20 minutes – so it was necessary to be selective about the topics that were included. We decided to focus on people's perceptions of communication, information, involvement and choice in health care.

A questionnaire was designed (see Appendix c) and NIPO, a Netherlands-based survey company, was asked to carry out interviews with 1000 people in each of the eight countries. The questionnaire was translated into the relevant languages and interviews were carried out in July 2002. The survey findings are outlined in Chapter 11.

International conference

The final results of the whole project were presented to an international audience at a conference held in Brussels in November 2002.

NOTES

1 Hensher, M., Fulop, N., Coast, J. and Jefferys, E. (2001) Better out than in? Alternatives to acute hospital care, *British Medical Journal*, **319**: 1127–30.

2 Goodwin, N. (1996) GP fundholding: a review of the evidence, *Health Care UK 1995/6*, pp. 116–30. London: King's Fund.

3 Figueras, J., Saltman, R.B. and Sakellarides, C. (1999) Introduction, in R.B. Saltman, J. Figueras and C. Sakellarides (eds) *Critical Challenges for Health Care Reform in Europe*, pp. 1–19. Buckingham: Open University Press, 1999.

4 Dixon, A. and Mossialos, E. (2001) Funding health care in Europe: recent experiences, *Health Care UK 2001*. London: King's Fund.

5 Anderson, G.F. and Poullier, J-P. (1999) Health spending, access, and outcomes: trends in industrialized countries, *Health Affairs*, **18**: 178–92.

6 Mossialos, E. (1998) *Citizens and Health Systems: Main Results from Eurobarometer Survey*. Geneva: European Commission Directorate General for Employment, Industrial Relations and Social Affairs.

7 Kutzin, J. (1999) The appropriate role for patient cost-sharing, in R.B. Saltman, J. Figueras and C. Sakellarides (eds) *Critical Challenges for Health Care Reform in Europe*, pp. 78–112. Buckingham: Open University Press.

8 Dargie, C., Dawson, S. and Garside, P. (2000) *Policy futures for UK health*. London: The Nuffield Trust and The Judge Institute of Management Studies, University of Cambridge.

9 Rosleff, F. and Lister, G. (1995) *European Healthcare Trends: Towards Managed Care in Europe*. Geneva: Coopers & Lybrand Europe Ltd.

10 Comptroller and Auditor General (2002) *NHS Direct in England*, HC505. London: The Stationery Office.

11 Peckham, M. (1998) Future health scenarios and public policy, in M. Marinker and M. Peckham (eds) *Clinical Futures*, pp. 184–209. London: BMJ Books.

12 European Commission, Directorate-General for Employment, Industrial Relations and Social Affairs (1999) *'Best Practice': State of the Art and Perspectives in the EU for improving the Effectiveness and Efficiency of European Health Systems*. Luxembourg: Office for Official Publications of the European Communities.

13 Durant, J. (1999) Public understanding of the significance of genomics, in

P. Williams and S. Clow (eds) *Genomics, Healthcare and Public Policy*, pp. 23–32. London: Office of Health Economics.

14 Bell, J. (1998) The human genome, in M. Marinker and M. Peckham (eds) *Clinical Futures*, pp. 20–42. London: BMJ Books.

15 Coulter, A., Entwistle, V. and Gilbert, D. (1999) Sharing decisions with patients: is the information good enough?, *British Medical Journal*, **318**: 318–22.

16 Wanless, D. (2002) *Securing Our Future Health: Taking a Long-term View* (final report). London: HM Treasury.

17 Coulter, A. (2002) *The Autonomous Patient*. London: Nuffield Trust.

18 Paton, C. (2002) *The Impact of Market Forces on Health Systems*. Dublin: European Health Management Association.

19 Vandenbroucke, F. (2002) The EU and social protection: what should the European Convention propose? Paper presented at the Max Planck Institute for the Study of Societies, Cologne, 17 June.

20 Coulter, A. and Ham, C. (2000) *The Global Challenge of Health Care Rationing*. Buckingham: Open University Press.

2

HEALTH SERVICES IN THE DIFFERENT COUNTRIES

THE STUDY COUNTRIES

European health systems share many characteristics, in particular the commitment to universal coverage, but they have adopted a diversity of organizational forms. Distinctions between the three main systems of funding – the Beveridge model based on taxation, the Bismarck model based on various forms of social insurance and the Eastern European Semashko model – are beginning to blur as successive reforms create a measure of convergence. Unfortunately it was not possible to study patients' experiences and expectations in all the countries in Europe, so eight were selected to represent the diversity of systems: Germany, Italy, Poland, Slovenia, Spain, Sweden, Switzerland and the United Kingdom. The key characteristics of their health systems are summarized in Table 2.1.

Germany

As Table 2.1 illustrates, the German health care system is relatively expensive – both in absolute terms and as a percentage of GDP. It is based on a statutory health insurance scheme with 10 per cent of the population being members of private insurance funds. Within this system, all those insured have free access to registered doctors, including specialists, and since 1996 most people have had the right to choose their sickness fund. It is a highly decentralized system with much of the responsibility delegated to the sickness funds and health care providers. There has traditionally been a clear separation between ambulatory care and hospital care. Ambulatory care has mainly been provided by private office-based physicians operating in solo practices with no gatekeeping role. Hospital treatment is provided by both public and private providers. The Reform Act of 2000 aimed to strengthen primary care, and reduce the separation between the ambulatory and in-patient sectors. Hospitals can now offer day surgery and pre and post in-patient care, and sickness funds were given the option of introducing gatekeeping systems on a voluntary basis.

The major objective of other recent reforms has been cost-containment. The Health Care Structure Act (1993) introduced more competition between sickness funds and in the hospital sector the First and Second SHI Restructuring Acts (1997/8) expanded market mechanisms and co-payments were increased. Despite these measures, the German health care system continues to spend money on a large number of providers and advanced medical technology. The public supports these priorities, and waiting lists and explicit rationing are virtually unknown.

Italy

Italy's health care system is financed by taxation and provides free universal coverage. But long waiting lists and regional variations in quality mean that an estimated 30 per cent of the population had private insurance in 1999, according to the European Observatory on Healthcare Systems.[1] Patient dissatisfaction remained high throughout the 1990s.

The recent reform process began in 1992 and is moving the health service towards a more decentralized system. The aim is to develop incentives for greater efficiency at both regional and local levels. Local health units were made self-governing public enterprises and their number reduced from 650 to 230, and larger specialist hospitals became independent agencies. In 2000 a law was passed which will eventually replace the national health fund with regional taxation. Regions unable to raise sufficient tax will be subsidized by central government. But one of the most striking features of the current situation is the inequality between regions, with standards of care lower in the south and central regions than in the north of the country. Another source of dissatisfaction is the high level of co-payments (see Table 2.1) and further reforms look to their gradual abolition. But despite the progress made in recent years there is still a great deal of uncertainty over the implementation of many of these reforms.

Table 2.1 Key health system characteristics of the eight selected countries

	Germany	Italy	Poland	Slovenia	Spain	Sweden	Switzerland	United Kingdom
Pop. (millions)	82	58	39	2	40	9	7	60
EU member?	Yes	Yes	No	No	Yes	Yes	No	Yes
Government	Red-green coalition (centre left, social democrat)	Multi-party coalition (conservative)	Democratic left alliance (centre left)	Coalition (social democrat, conservative)	Centre right popular party	Social democrat	Coalition (centre right, social and Christian democrat)	Labour (centre left, social democrat)
Life expectancy (at birth) in 1999	Males: 73.7 (a) Females: 80.1 (a)	Males: 75.4 (a) Females: 82.1 (a)	Males: 68.8(i) Females: 77.5 (i)	Males: 71.6 (a) Females: 79.5 (a)	Males: 75.3 (a) Females: 82.1 (a)	Males: 76.2(a) Females: 81.4 (a)	Males: 75.6 (a) Females: 83.0 (a)	Males: 74.7 (a) Females: 79.7 (a)
Leading causes of death	Circulatory diseases, cancer	Circulatory diseases, cancer	Circulatory diseases, cancer	Circulatory diseases, cancer	Circulatory diseases, cancer	Circulatory diseases, cancer	Circulatory diseases, cancer	Circulatory diseases, cancer
Health system	Regional with national legal framework	Regional with national legal framework	Regional with national legal framework	Centrally administered with moves towards decentralization of primary care	Centrally funded, centrally and regionally administered	Regional with national legal framework	Regional with national legal framework	NHS centrally funded and administered

% of GDP spent on health care in 2000	10.6 (b)	8.1 (b)	6.2 (1999) (b)	7.7 (1999) (c)	7.7 (b)	7.9 (1998) (b)	10.7 (b)	7.3 (b)
Total per capita spending (in US$) in 2000	2748 (b)	2032 (b)	507 (1999) (b)	1101 (1998) (c)	1556 (b)	1748 (1998) (b)	3222 (b)	1763 (b)
Public expenditure as % of total spending in 2000	75.1 (b)	73.7 (b)	75.1 (1999) (b)	86.0 (c)	69.9 (b)	83.8 (1998) (b)	55.6 (b)	81.0 (b)
Funding mechanism	Social insurance	Taxation	Social insurance taking over from government funding	Compulsory health insurance	Taxation	Decentralized taxation	Social insurance and taxation	Taxation
Purchasers/commissioners	453 sickness insurance funds and 52 private insurers	199 local health authorities	Health insurance funds taking over from government	National Health Insurance Institute	Purchaser/provider split not yet implemented	18 county councils, 2 regions, 1 municipality	26 cantons, 109 insurance companies	300 primary care trusts in England, health boards in Scotland, Wales and Northern Ireland

Table 2.1—*continued*

	Germany	Italy	Poland	Slovenia	Spain	Sweden	Switzerland	United Kingdom
Providers	Single-handed ambulatory care physicians (GPs and specialists), 2081 general hospitals, 33 teaching hospitals, 207 psychiatric hospitals	Independent contracted GPs, acute and rehabilitation hospitals, public hospital trusts, private accredited providers	8227 health care institutions, 715 general hospitals	64 health care centres, 62 health care stations, 26 general, specialist and clinical hospitals, 16 spas (h)	2500 health centres, 3334 health posts, 799 hospitals (public and private)	Salaried GPs, 950 health centres, regional, central and district county hospitals, private hospitals	3792 individual practices, health maintenance organizations, 226 general and 180 specialist hospitals (public, subsidized and private)	Independent contracted GPs, NHS Trusts running hospitals, primary care, mental health and ambulance services, private hospitals
Out-of-pocket as % of total health spending	11.3 (a)	41.8 (a)	28.4 (a)	10.2 (a)	20.4 (a)	22.0 (a)	29.7 (a)	3.1 (a)
No. of practising physicians per 1000 pop. in 2000	3.6 (b)	6.0 (b)	2.2 (b)	2.2 (1999) (c)	3.3 (b)	2.9 (1999) (b)	3.5 (b)	1.8 (b)
No. of nurses per 1000 pop.	9.5 (1999) (c)	5.3 (1997) (b)	5.1 (1999) (i)	6.9 (1999) (h)	5.1 (1998) (c)	8.2 (1997) (c)	7.8 (1990) (c)	5.0 (1998) (b)

	Direct	Via GP	Via GP (although sometimes bypassed)	Via GP	Via GP for most	Via GP except for paediatrics, gynaecology, psychiatry	Direct to ambulatory specialists	Via GP
Access to specialists	Direct	Via GP	Via GP (although sometimes bypassed)	Via GP	Via GP for most	Via GP except for paediatrics, gynaecology, psychiatry	Direct to ambulatory specialists	Via GP
Total inpatient care beds per 1000 pop. in 2000	9.1 (b)	4.9 (1999) (c)	4.9 (b)	5.4 acute (1999) (h)	4.1 (b)	3.6 (b)	17.9 (b)	4.1 (b)
Average length of acute hospital stay in 2000	9.6 days (b)	7.2 days (1998) (b)	9.3 days (1999) (i)	7.6 days (1999) (c)	8.5 days (1998)(c)	5 days (b)	9.3 days (b)	6.2 (b)
Patients' rights	Many patient groups but political arm absent. Reform Act 2000 strengthens patients' rights. Patients' Charter published but not legally binding	Article 32 of constitution guarantees right to health. From 1980 about 80 Patients' Charters proposed. 1994 Health Services Charters introduced.	1991 Health Care Institutions Act enshrined patients' rights. Charter of Patients' Rights being developed	Article 51 of 1995 Constitution lists the right to health care as fundamental. Citizens may participate directly in parliamentary health care debates and on regional committees of the insured	Citizens' participation incorporated into General Health Care Act 1986 but user groups weak. 1994 Charter on Rights and Duties	Patients' rights spread over 20–25 different laws and decrees. 1997 Official document: *The Patient is Right*. 1999 Patients' Rights Reform increased county councils' obligations	Patients' organizations work on various committees but patients' rights vary from canton to canton. Law passed in canton of Geneva in late 1980s supporting patients' rights	Patients' Charter 1991 set national standards but is not legally binding. Independent Patients' Association, numerous self-help groups

Table 2.1—*continued*

	Germany	Italy	Poland	Slovenia	Spain	Sweden	Switzerland	United Kingdom
Internet users 2000	19.1m (e)	11.6m (e)	6.1m (j)	300,000 (1998) (f)	5.2m (e)	3.5 (e)	2.0 (2001) (g)	17.9m (e)

Notes:
a: World Health Report 2000
b: OECD Health Data 2002
c: WHO Regional Office for Europe
d: European Observatory on Health Care Systems
e: Computer Industry Almanac
f: Research on the Internet in Slovenia
g: Jupiter Media Matrix
h: Health Statistics Yearbook, Slovenia 1999
i: Statistical Yearbook of the Republic of Poland, 2000
j: Demoskop Survey Oct. 2000

Poland

The Polish health care system has undergone significant changes since 1989 when the political and economic transformation of the country began. In 1999 a health service controlled and financed by the state was replaced by a new health insurance scheme. The previous financing method had relied on transferring money to medical institutions on an historic budgetary principle unrelated to productivity. The new method of funding involves transferring money from health premiums to 16 regional sick funds. Each fund operates independently in shaping the product it pays for, as well as in terms of the rates and limits of contracted services.

Unwieldy infrastructures are common problems in the health systems of Eastern Europe and Poland is no exception. Total spending on health is much less than in the other countries in this study (see Table 2.1). Health care reforms were introduced in parallel with other major reforms in social security and education but they have received the most criticism. Universal access has been maintained but equity is increasingly under threat in a system where low salaries among health professionals fuel extensive informal payments, making care unaffordable for a significant proportion of the population. A new family doctor service with a gatekeeping role has been established. Hospital care is being rationalized through regulation and reduced capacity, but the management of the new system is still in the very early stages of development.

Slovenia

The political upheavals in Eastern Europe in the late 1980s and early 1990s had major repercussions for health services in the region. Slovenia declared independence on 25 June 1991 and health care reform was one of the first important changes. The Healthcare and Health Insurance Act (1992) established the present system of compulsory and voluntary health insurance and introduced privatization. New medical and pharmaceutical chambers took over much of the administration of the system and in 1999 a new mutual health insurance organization was established to manage voluntary health insurance. Primary care is delivered by publicly owned health care centres and units. Secondary care is provided by hospitals, clinics and private specialists.

The private insurance sector has grown more quickly than anticipated and this has enabled Slovenia to offset some of the effects of the declining revenues experienced elsewhere in Eastern Europe. Thus, although Slovenia spends less than the Western European countries in this study, its total per capita spending is still twice that of Poland (see Table 2.1). On the downside, some people fear that private insurance, together with cost-containment measures like the introduction of co-payments and a reduced benefits package, may undermine the equity achieved under the communist system.

Spain

In the last two decades, the Spanish health system – like other political and social institutions – has been going through a major process of transformation. The implementation of the General Health Law approved by Parliament in 1986 meant that free universal health coverage became a reality for all Spanish citizens. This law also laid the foundations for the national health system and led to the progressive devolution of health management to the autonomous communities or regional governments. To date, decentralization has been implemented in 7 of the 17 communities.

The health service is funded from general taxation, collected by central government and allocated to the communities on a per capita basis. Additional sources of finance come from out-of-pocket payments and private voluntary insurance that covers 10 per cent of the population.

Rising costs and low levels of public satisfaction have driven recent reforms. There has been an extensive reform of the primary care sector and 60 new public hospitals have been built. The first Central Health Plan (1995) set 14 priority areas for action including the elderly, AIDS, cancer and mental health. From January 2000, patients waiting more than six months had the right to choose another hospital.

But devolution makes overall cost containment difficult and different rates of public expenditure in the regions have created variations in health care standards. Another major problem is the difficulty of gathering information and coordinating services across the regions.

Sweden

The Swedish health care system is a regionally based, publicly financed and, to a very high degree, publicly provided national

health service. Responsibility for most health care planning and provision has been decentralized from the national level to the county
councils and the municipalities who own and manage hospitals and
health centres.

The Swedes enjoy some of the highest living standards in the
world and Sweden's health care system has traditionally provided
good access to high quality services. Only a very small minority
take out private insurance and the central government sets a ceiling
on out-of-pocket payments. But as elsewhere in Europe, economic
pressure in the 1980s and 1990s led to demands for cost containment and an expansion of the private sector. The recent reforms
have attempted to address these issues but the highly decentralized
nature of the system has made a coordinated strategy difficult and
progress has been uneven across the counties. On the other hand,
increasing cost awareness has led to more cooperation between the
counties.

There is evidence that the changes have also led to a decrease
in patient satisfaction. There have been reductions in staffing levels
and waiting times have increased. The main challenges in the future
will be to balance the need for greater cost effectiveness with the
traditionally high expectations of patients who are becoming more
vocal and influential.

Switzerland

Switzerland has a rather complex health system for a country with
just over 7 million inhabitants. It is governed by laws on health care
insurance at the federal level, which provide the basis for equality of
access across the country. But the system is mainly managed at the
level of the cantons – the 26 units of local government. In addition,
the country has three main linguistic groups: German (65 per cent),
French (18 per cent) and Italian (10 per cent). Variations in wealth,
culture and politics explain some of the striking differences and
inequalities between the cantons.

Health services are funded primarily through compulsory
health insurance schemes subsidized by taxation. Co-payments
and direct out-of-pocket payments are relatively high as not all
services are included in the benefits package, although these are
being expanded.

In absolute terms, Switzerland spends more on health than any
other country in our study and also enjoys the highest hospital
density and one of the highest doctor-patient ratios (see Table 2.1).

But the traditionally decentralized system, in which providers can choose where to locate and patients can choose providers within their own canton, is changing. Federal government powers are increasing and managed care systems are being established in an attempt to cut costs and control spending on out-patient care and pharmaceuticals. It remains to be seen whether patients who pay dearly for their health service will be prepared to accept these measures.

United Kingdom

The National Health Service (NHS) provides health care largely free at the point of delivery. National taxation is the main source of funding although co-payments are charged for certain drugs and services and a minority of the population (about 13 per cent) has private insurance. The percentage of gross domestic product (GDP) spent on health care is somewhat lower than most of the other countries in this study (see Table 2.1) but it has been increasing under the current Labour government. Multi-disciplinary teams based in local health centres provide most of the primary care services. Publicly-owned hospital trusts are the main provider of secondary care.

Elements of the earlier reforms carried out under the Conservative government in the 1990s have been retained – for example, the purchaser/provider split. But more recent changes aim to replace competition within the internal market by collaboration and partnership. The UK has traditionally had a strong primary care sector and the creation of new primary care trusts (PCTs) has reinforced this. They provide both primary and community health services and are in the process of becoming the main purchasers of health care.

Health policy and the quality of health care is very high on the political agenda. Two new agencies – the National Institute of Clinical Excellence (NICE) and the Commission for Health Improvement – have been established to raise standards, a Modernization Board has been set up to oversee changes, and 26 health action zones have been created to improve the health of deprived populations. But waiting lists remain the public's main cause for concern and many remain unconvinced that the government can deliver the improvements it has promised.

SIMILARITIES AND DIFFERENCES

Funding

The health systems in the eight countries included in this study differ in a number of important respects. In four – Italy, Spain, Sweden and the UK – health care is funded primarily out of taxation, while in the other four – Germany, Poland, Slovenia and Switzerland – social insurance is the primary funding mechanism. Germany and Switzerland spend more than 10 per cent of their GDP on health care while the other countries spend between 6 and 8 per cent. Spending levels also differ in absolute terms with the highest, Switzerland, spending about six times more dollars per capita than the lowest, Poland.

Comparisons of the impact of different funding levels are not straightforward because costs differ, but staffing levels vary dramatically. For example, Italy has three times more practising doctors per head of population than the UK, and Germany has nearly twice as many nurses as Italy, Poland, Spain and the UK. Provision of hospital beds ranges from 17.9 per 1000 population in Switzerland to 3.6 in Sweden, but this reflects differences in patterns of admission and discharge. For example, more care is provided outside hospital for Swedish patients where the average length of inpatient stay is only five days, as compared to nearly ten days in Germany. Variations in rates of out-of-pocket spending are even more dramatic, with Italian patients making financial contributions to their health care at more than ten times the rate of British patients.

Devolution

Health care is administered differently in each of the countries. The systems are highly decentralized in Germany, Sweden and Switzerland, with funding and authority located at regional levels, but centrally administered by national authorities in the UK and Slovenia. In most countries the trend appears to be going towards greater devolution of power. Spain and Italy are currently undergoing transitions from a centrally to a locally administered system and elements of devolution are being introduced in Slovenia. A process of devolution is also under way in the UK, where primary care trusts are taking over budgetary responsibility for the care of local residents. Meanwhile in Switzerland, where responsibility for health care has long been devolved to the cantons, the federal government is increasing its power and influence. Indeed, at the same time as speeding up the decentralization of administrative responsibility, most countries are in the process of establishing or strengthening national bodies to take responsibility for overseeing professional training, regulation and quality assurance.

Gatekeeping

The balance between primary and secondary care also varies, with different degrees of freedom of choice for patients about who they can consult. The UK has a relatively strong primary care system in which patients register with a GP and cannot access specialist services (except in emergencies or other special circumstances) without a GP referral. Patients in Italy, Slovenia, Spain and Sweden are also expected to register with local GPs or other physicians working in primary care – for example, paediatricians – and use them for first contact care, and Poland has just introduced a similar gatekeeping system. Patients in Germany and Switzerland can consult specialists directly if they wish without being referred by a GP.

Gatekeeping or managed care systems are generally perceived to be more efficient and the authorities in those countries that lack these systems are making various attempts to introduce them on a voluntary basis. In Germany, attempts are being made to strengthen primary care and gatekeeping systems are being introduced by some sickness funds, while in Switzerland managed care systems are being introduced in an attempt to control spending on ambulatory care and pharmaceuticals. In the meantime, the UK has introduced nurse-led 'walk-in' centres aimed at providing more flexible access and relieving the pressure on hospital emergency departments.

Patients' rights

Legislation to protect patients' rights exists in each of the countries and the last decade has seen various attempts to strengthen this, often by introducing patients' charters. For the most part these are simply statements or clarifications of existing rights and entitlements, designed to increase awareness among patients and health care providers, rather than new primary legislation. Other initiatives to empower patients have included provision of health information and education about prevention, establishment of advice centres and helplines, official support and funding for patients' groups, and public consultation and opportunities to participate in debates about health policy.

Managing demand

Despite the differences in structure, funding and organization, all countries' health systems are facing similar pressures and cost drivers. Demographic trends mean that people are living longer and the costs of chronic disease management and long-term care are rising. Policy makers have to respond to these trends. Examples of initiatives taken in one or more of the eight countries include structural reforms designed to control costs and promote greater efficiency, such as hospital mergers or the introduction of primary care gatekeeping systems; attempts to strengthen the funding base by reforming funding mechanisms, increasing out-of-pocket payments or introducing incentives to encourage private investment; reassessment of professional responsibilities and encouragement of extended roles for nurses, pharmacists and other professional staff aimed at achieving better value for money; and the introduction of new, potentially faster routes of access to health advice – for example, by the provision of health websites, telephone and email consultations or telemedicine.

New technologies are being developed and promoted commercially and policy makers have to decide whether to concede to pressures to extend the scope of reimbursable medical care to include such things as alternative and complementary therapies, new medicines designed for previously 'untreatable' conditions or self-diagnosis kits and genetic screening. Patients' demands for more information about diseases, treatments and services, greater involvement in treatment decisions, more support for self-care and increased choice of providers and treatments also require a response from policy makers.

Public confidence

Above all, European governments have to ensure that social consensus remains intact and policy developments are in tune with wider social values. It is seen as important that citizens and the electorate understand the basis of health care reforms and feel informed about policy changes and their underlying justification. In several of our study countries there have been recent initiatives to secure greater public involvement in policy debates as policy makers attempt to ensure that any restrictions on the growth and availability of health services strike an acceptable balance in the eyes of the public as legitimate trade-offs between the supply of services and the expenditure of public funds.

Despite the differences, these countries are facing similar challenges – principally, increased costs brought about by an ageing population, increased availability of new treatments and technology, and rising public expectations. At the same time, patients are no longer willing to remain passive participants and are demanding greater choice and more involvement in decision making. For a number of reasons, therefore, these countries are re-examining the structure of their health systems. In Eastern Europe, reforms have been triggered by political change, and in Western Europe by a need to contain rising costs and increase efficiency.

Given the diversity and complexity of the health systems, this relatively small-scale study of patients' views and experiences in eight countries cannot hope to provide definitive answers to the policy makers' dilemma. But by comparing and contrasting the case studies, drawing out the similarities as well as the differences, a more comprehensive picture begins to emerge of the likely response of European patients to future trends in health care.

ADDITIONAL SOURCES

Abel-Smith, B., Figueras, J., Holland, W., McKee, M. and Mossialos, E. (1995) *Choices in Health Care Policy*. Aldershot: Dartmouth Publishing Company.

Freeman, R. (2000) *The Politics of Health in Europe*. Manchester: Manchester University Press.

Mattison, N. (2000) *Patients' Rights: Global Overview*. Princeton, N.J.: The Mattison Group.

Saltman, R.B., Figueras, J. and Sakellarides, C. (eds) (1998) *Critical Challenges for Health Care Reform in Europe*. Buckingham: Open University Press.

3

GERMANY

OPINIONS ABOUT THE HEALTH CARE SYSTEM

The present system

The German health care system is financed by statutory health insurance. Ninety per cent of the population is insured against the risk of sickness on a statutory basis, the other 10 per cent are members of private insurance funds. All insured persons have free access to registered doctors, including specialist consultants, and efforts to restrict this would find no majority support at the moment.[1] A chip card (or smart card) is issued by sickness funds to all their members. It confirms their insured status and they show it whenever they enter a surgery or hospital. It also means that patients do not need a referral document to contact a specialist and is considered a very important instrument of individual choice.

In the eyes of its users, the German health care system has proved itself even during periods of economic downturn (almost 30 per cent are fully behind this statement, while 54 per cent express qualified support).[2] The majority of the population considers statutory health insurance, including the principle of solidarity and the free health insurance of members of the insured's family, to be adequate (93 per cent). This applies across all population groups and all ages.[2,3,4]

Access and responsiveness

There are no restrictions on access to health care facilities in the outpatient sector, and any insured person has the right to seek out a registered doctor of his or her choice. The physician density in

Germany is high: in 1997 there were 345 doctors per 100,000 population. If people need hospital care the next two reachable hospitals suitable for the planned treatment must be specified when a referral is made. If individuals choose a hospital other than one of those specified in the doctor's referral without a good reason, the supplementary costs could be charged to them in part or in total. The same principle applies to the reimbursement of travelling expenses.[5]

While waiting lists are not a problem in the German system (not a single person in the group discussions talked about these), people did complain about waiting times in clinics: *'I think everyone can wait half an hour but if I'm at the specialist's and there's an emergency every time, then I can't believe it any more'.*

The German system is not without problems. On the one hand, the largely equal access to services, the high number of doctors, beds, medicines and therapeutic aids available, the high level of research spending and a favourable ranking in birth mortality rates are all testimony to good quality. On the other hand, Germany achieves only a middle ranking in terms of life expectancy in comparison to other Organization for Economic Cooperation and Development (OECD) countries, a middle ranking in avoidable deaths for coronary heart disease, rising mortality from intestinal and breast cancer,[6] and only a middle ranking in terms of patient satisfaction in an international comparison.[7] There are also regional differences – for example in the mortality rates in the new and old federal Lander.[8]

According to the results of representative population surveys, 74 per cent of Germans are satisfied with their health care system and care facilities, while their faith in doctors remains high.[2] Nevertheless, when people who had frequent contact with health care organizations were surveyed, an extensive list of shortcomings emerged, from a lack of openness about treatment information and standards, to long diagnosis times, too little knowledge of the latest status of research and lack of coordination.[9] There is potential for improvement in the representation of patients' interests and in the management of complaints in hospitals. A lack of caring attention is especially complained about. In hospital, about two thirds of patients feel they are treated more as a number than as a person or even a customer.[1]

It became obvious in the focus group discussions that a high level of distrust about the quality of the health service coexisted with apparent satisfaction with the system and individual doctors. This distrust was based on patients' own experiences and the experiences of relatives, friends and colleagues. It was also exacerbated by a sense of injustice because the economic interests of physicians have led to increases in co-payments for diagnostic and therapeutic procedures.

Nearly all participants in the focus groups felt the role of the physician had changed in recent years. Increasingly they were seen as having to balance their health care tasks with their business and financial interests, as well as dealing with the legal and financial restrictions of limited health care budgets: *'My GP told me that if this recession goes too far, he won't be able to treat me any more, because I'm simply too expensive for him. And he is not the only one. It seems to be the rule in our city that chronically ill patients are consciously treated in an unfriendly manner, they don't get the drugs they need'.*

Participants talked about physicians who closed their offices in the second third of the month, claiming that the budget was used up: *'He says: I do not work for nothing, I shut up shop'.*

Patients with chronic conditions complained of lack of co-operation between sickness funds and physicians: *'If I go to the health insurance fund, they say: We provide this for you. However, the doctor blocks it. When I go to the doctor, he says: I would prescribe this or that for you with pleasure but the fund doesn't allow it'.*

Structure and organization

Almost everybody has their own GP. Having a GP is accepted in principle: *'The central issue is that you find a good GP, in fact a doctor whom you can trust, where you have the feeling that you are in good hands'.* Patients who have found a doctor they trust do not usually change doctors, even if they are not satisfied with the organization of the practice and have to suffer long waiting times.[1,10]

The most recent legal regulations promote the principle of the family doctor as gatekeeper. The health insurance institutions can offer a bonus for individuals who voluntarily use family doctors as gatekeepers, thus limiting their freedom to use outpatient medical services. The transition to the voluntary family doctor system envisaged by the legislature is intended to achieve cost reductions.[11]

The new role of GPs as gatekeepers in the health care system is controversial. The freedom to choose a doctor was talked about again and again, and defended as an important principle: *'I would like to have the possibility to consult a specialist directly if I know what I have. When I have back pain, I do not need to consult my GP to be referred to the specialist'.*

Some participants felt the gatekeeper model increases the cost of health care, while others felt it decreases it:

In my opinion that is very expensive. If I use this example – I first go to my GP, he examines me, then he writes a referral, and then I go with my sprained foot to the orthopaedist, to whom I could have gone right from the start. That is double the cost.

I think specialists are relatively expensive, and when I'm treated there it is certainly more expensive than if the house doctor does it.

It was repeatedly pointed out by participants that the gatekeeper model puts the GP in a powerful position.

Cost and efficiency

Debate about the financing of the health care system centres on the stability of the contributions paid into the statutory scheme. Control is exercised through budgets in the inpatient and outpatient sectors as well as in the area of medication, but supplementary fees (e.g. in the case of medicines or hospital stays) are also relevant. Patients can be affected in different ways by these controls, particularly chronically sick patients who experience restrictions on prescriptions. Such experiences lead to diminishing faith in the performance of statutory health insurance schemes and also to a sense of a 'two-tier system'.[12] Most people say that they would be willing to pay higher contributions in order to safeguard the level of care, but 80 per cent think that a great deal of money is wasted in the health system.[3]

Certain services are no longer financed by statutory health insurance schemes and patients are expected to make supplementary payments. For example, treatments for the common cold, influenza, constipation and travel sickness, plus some screening programmes, are no longer covered by statutory health insurance schemes. Health costs incurred by private households amounted to DM34.2 billion in 1994. This represents 10 per cent of health costs. In 1994, 56 per cent of private health spending went on goods (medication, medical aids and dentures), 21 per cent went on therapeutic services, while 11 per cent was spent on hotel services in hospitals and facilities for preventive care, rehabilitation and nursing. A further 10 per cent was spent on physicians' and dentists' services, including treatments associated with dentures.[13]

Focus group participants were worried about financial develop-ments: '*What I simply don't understand is why one pays a bigger and bigger contribution for smaller and smaller benefits*'.

Participants felt a new customer-salesperson relationship has developed between doctors and patients. Some doctors display price lists for self-financed supplementary services in their waiting rooms. This emphasizes the impression that while doctors are recommending preventive services for the care of the patient, they are also selling their products and taking care of themselves financially. It is interesting to see that patients develop their own strategies to deal with this situation. They use screening (for example mammography), but claim to have symptoms or pain so the diagnostic procedure is paid for by the sickness fund. Participants talked about doctors who demanded money for procedures that should have been a regular part of the consultation: '*There was a sheet of paper on the counter that said if I talk to this GP for more than ten minutes in three months, I will get a private bill*'.

Supplementary payments have now reached such dimensions that talk of a second health insurance contribution seems justified. At present, a general upper limit applies (modified for chronically sick patients) of 2 per cent of a person's annual gross income. For a patient who is not self-employed, this figure implies in extreme cases a rise of around 30 per cent in health costs. Older people, the disabled and the chronically ill are particularly affected by the additional contribution arrangements:

> *For the chronically ill person it is horrendously expensive. A per-son who is not chronically ill does not have the high consumption of medicines that we do and the more serious the disease the more we have to pay, and for those who are handicapped through the illness and perhaps unable to work, they are in a very bad financial situation, because they need their medicine, and if they don't get it, they have a hard time. So it's a vicious cycle.*

In fact, there are some exemptions and lots of ways to reduce the financial burden but not all patients know about these rules and procedures.

Equity

In spite of increasing costs, the health insurance system with its solidarity principle was supported by the majority of participants, in particular by those with chronic diseases. A few people questioned whether contribution-free family health insurance should be maintained: *'For children I am absolutely ready to pay. However, not for wives who don't work'.*

The majority of participants were satisfied in terms of value for money but most of them were convinced that the scope of the social safety net would not be sustainable at this level in the future. Some participants approved of the idea that unhealthy or risky lifestyles could lead to higher contribution rates, particularly as part of strengthening people's direct responsibility and saving costs. For example, on the question of treatment for alcoholism, one participant said: *'Therefore if someone asked me, I wouldn't be willing to pay extra in my contribution because I do not drink. People shouldn't drink so much'.*

However, all participants saw the definition of a 'risk group' as particularly crucial. The conversion to a higher insurance contribution for people with high risk lifestyles fails at a practical level because the dividing line between high and low risk is very blurred: *'It begins with certain types of sport, then smoker or non-smoker, and people who are too fat. Where does it end? One day if you only eat a few cucumbers you're considered to live the wrong way'.*

Some people were happy to pay a higher contribution rate to have better care: *'I like the idea that for example one pays DM20 more per month and you get more and you can use alternative medicines'.*

Only a few people accepted the idea of separation into optional and basic services in the statutory health insurance schemes: *'I would be ready to pay a little separately, then I would have this extra safety-net, which I do not have now'.* However, some of those consulted recognized these tendencies already: *'In any case very strong trends are evident . . . some people top up their individual insurance with extra cover depending on their financial possibilities'.* New insurance schemes require highly informed users. They have to decide *'. . . what I want to protect and what not'.*

However, optional and basic services should be clearly defined, otherwise it was felt there would be a danger that health insurers could refuse to pay for life-saving treatment and the community would have to fulfil this obligation. The social consequences of differentiation were perceived clearly by participants who feared the development of a two-tier health system: *'But there are sick people who cannot afford it. What should they do? They must bite the dust'.*

PATIENTS' VIEWS OF HEALTH PROFESSIONALS

Doctors

Focus group participants felt that information and communication between doctor and patient were the most important indicators of good health care, followed by knowledge of complaint procedures, face-to-face consultations or continuity of care. Another important aspect of good health care for the group participants was access to different treatment options, and particularly to complementary therapies and medicines. It was felt that sickness funds should be ready to pay for these.

Complete and utter trust in doctors was expressed by 20 per cent of those polled in one survey.[2] Only around 20 per cent of Germans said they had little or no trust in GPs. The health care system permits the user to 'try out' a doctor. In doing this, patients assume their role as customers and can terminate an unsatisfactory doctor-patient relationship if they choose. They change doctors when they are dissatisfied with what for them are important aspects of treatment or practice management.[14] A survey conducted among 1100 parents caring for asthmatic children showed, for example, that only one third of parents found a doctor at first try who, in their eyes, initiated effective therapy, while another third visited three or more doctors before they felt that their child was treated properly.[15]

Nearly all participants were satisfied with their own physician, even if they quoted numerous negative examples from former experiences. The most frequent criticism was the lack of time and attention for the individual patient. An example given by a young man illustrates this: '*I came in and was told quickly what I had. He didn't allow me to express my view, and immediately I got a notification of illness and a prescription, before I could say anything. Doctors don't take care of their patients, they don't listen*'.

Generally speaking, people would like doctors to talk to them more and prescribe less, and they are not completely satisfied with the emotional care and attention they receive and the time taken by doctors in consultations.[2]

Nevertheless, in the first instance, the general level of confidence in the medical profession was high among all groups, including the younger participants: '*I basically go to the doctor in the hope that he can help me and that I can trust him too. And I don't start by distrusting him*'.

Nurses

Almost three quarters of those polled in a population study considered doctors, nurses and carers to be overburdened.[2] Attitudes towards nurses varied in the focus groups, with both good and bad experiences reported. Some participants saw nurses as highly competent professionals, while others emphasized their poor vocational training. Most saw them simply as doctors' assistants and not as professionals with their own responsibilities. An extension of nurses' role was considered possible by some participants but others, particularly women, disapproved of the idea: *'I would not have great confidence in them. They have a completely different training'*. On the other hand, participants had already witnessed an increase in nurses' responsibilities: *'I think nurses do have more responsibility in fact. When you go to some specialists, it is often the nurse who carries out the preliminary diagnosis and the doctor only comes in to make the final diagnosis'*. It seems that people are beginning to accept these developments, *'The nurse is also trained in medical things, to diagnose a sprained foot or a sprained wrist, to see whether it's sprained or broken. Why not? For simple things, this is all right'* and in some cases nurses were regarded as more competent than physicians: *'... so some nurses know more or are more qualified in specific things than the doctor'*.

The financial advantages of expanding the nurse's role were mentioned: *'A nurse does not cost as much as a doctor, and so we could have more of them and that way the waiting period could be reduced, and the GP would only have to deal with those things which only he can decide on'*. However, as a precondition for increasing the nurse's role, participants felt they would require further training, regular monitoring, and clinical specialization – for example, the 'rheumatism nurse' or the nurse for the elderly: *'If I had a nurse with a specialization in rheumatology who could also prescribe medicines, I would not have any problems with this'*.

Participants felt there was a risk of potential conflict between nurses and physicians and there was a feeling that diagnosis should always stay within the physicians' jurisdiction. Liability issues should be clarified. If the responsibilities of nurses are to be increased, this should be matched with more training and further education.

Pharmacists

Pharmacists are the first port of call for minor ailments and the over-the-counter market is increasing. Information provided by pharmacists was appreciated and used by focus group participants. Pharmacists were considered to be customer-oriented and they have enough time to give detailed information: *'Doctors don't like to give detailed explanations, and that is not true for the pharmacists. They speak my language, I understand it'*. In addition, pharmacists can act as a control mechanism, checking the prescriptions of physicians: *'. . . and then there would be a pharmacist who considers whether what the doctor prescribed is correct, or are there any mistakes due to the dosage or something like that'*.

But participants were ambivalent about increasing the pharmacist's responsibilities. Arguments in favour of widening their role included the good service they provide and a reduction of time spent in the doctor's surgery, as patients could go directly to the pharmacist instead of having a prescription from their physician: *'Sometimes it is also much easier when you go into a pharmacy – you are dealt with in five minutes, but if you go to the doctor, you have to wait for hours'*.

Pharmacists could also provide cheaper medicines. However, participants also raised concerns. Pharmacists are dependent on their sales figures. More opportunities to prescribe and more over-the-counter medicines could lead to economically motivated recommendations and a situation where prescriptions were influenced by financial considerations rather than concern for the patient: *'He is also a businessman, and in this respect he advises according to the medicines he wants to sell'*.

ALTERNATIVE WAYS OF ACCESSING HEALTH ADVICE

Telephone

Health insurance agencies in Germany have increasingly been offering their members free general health advice over the telephone. The long-term aim of these services is to develop telephone-supported disease management programmes for their insured. In addition there are commercial service providers who disseminate health information in return for fees or membership of an association.

Only a few focus group participants had sought health advice over the telephone, but people liked the idea of having quick and easy access to experts for a given health problem: *'I like this idea. I think it is good to make a call rather than going to the doctor. I do not go to see the doctor often. I have no time for that'*.

People valued the fact that telephone services are also easy to reach at the weekend or at night, and that they can contact a specialist if they feel worried about health problems: *'Then one can reach for the telephone and say: What do you say with regard to that? Or reassuring patients, that can also be done by telephone'*. However, it was felt that only very general information could be given on the phone, owing to legal restrictions.

Telemedicine

Germany is not very advanced in the area of telemedicine.[16] In accordance with the doctors' professional code, remote diagnosis without direct (physical) contact between doctor and patient is not yet permitted in Germany, but changes can be expected in the future. German-language advisory services located abroad are already on offer via the internet, and these services largely escape controls within the country.

Focus group participants were rather sceptical about the use of telemedicine, perhaps because they had little experience of it. Most preferred direct contact with a doctor. Telemedicine was seen as a complement to, rather than a substitute for, direct doctor-patient contact: *'I would approve of it for older people who can't walk very well or who need regular examinations'*. It was also seen as being potentially useful for those living in rural areas: *'If you are somewhere in Aurich or in the country somewhere in Eastern Friesland and you would have to travel 50km to see your doctor, then you might think about telemedicine'*.

Participants welcomed the notion that new technologies would enable consultation with the best doctors anywhere in the world and specialists would be able to treat patients regardless of their location.

EXTENDING THE SCOPE OF MEDICAL CARE

Complementary therapies

Three alternative therapies (phytotherapy, anthroposophy and homeopathy) form part of the physician's contractual services in

Germany. Many different types of complementary therapies are covered by individual health insurance schemes. Of those surveyed, 65 per cent used natural remedies at least once in 1997,[17] and 84 per cent of Germans would like to see more extensive use of natural methods in medicine.[18] This resort to complementary therapies is seen as a criticism of conventional medicine and of the health system.

Some focus group participants were concerned about the training of complementary practitioners: *'If I consider how you can become a naturopath today, about dubious distance learning courses, I start doubting'*.

There were a variety of views on how the costs of alternative treatments should be covered by the sickness funds. In most cases patients have to pay for themselves and participants felt this was unfair.

New medicines and biotechnologies

The willingness of people to use new technologies such as genetic screening can only be estimated at the moment. The main concern expressed in the focus groups was about how patients would cope with genetic information and whether effective treatments are available for the illnesses diagnosed:[19] *'It would be interesting if one knew the situation and was able to prevent the illness. If not, I would find it rather depressing and a burden'*.

Doubts were expressed about the wisdom of being screened for genetic susceptibility to cancer when treatment is still uncertain: *'Imagine the danger if cancer is in your genes. I would go mad knowing that'; 'Gene investigation in order to understand or cure illnesses, that's fine, however, it is not OK to manipulate human beings'*.

It was felt important that genetic tests should be voluntary. Freedom of choice must be guaranteed: *'To make it an obligation would be fatal. To have the choice, however, is completely appropriate'*.

The participants considered what interests employers would have in testing their prospective employees. Some were sympathetic to the needs of employers: *'I can absolutely understand that the employer would like to know that if I am offered a high-paid job, I'll be able to stick to it'*. But the majority thought that this kind of information should not be accessible to employers. Participants also saw problems in relation to data protection. If the results were made available to health insurers, for example, people predisposed to a given disease might be refused insurance because of the financial risks to the sickness fund: '*If you live in America, you do not have any health insurance. They do not insure you with this type of result'*.

Some younger participants were concerned about the cost of genetic screening and called for cost-benefit analyses comparing the costs of the tests against the benefits of disease prevention.

INFORMATION FOR PATIENTS

Health information needs

In a survey of around 1000 patients aged 18 to 80 in practices run by GPs and specialists, 93 per cent of those polled rated information as 'very important'. However, only 50 per cent of those patients were 'very satisfied' with the information received.[20] Another survey of 30,000 patients from 450 practices in Berlin also showed an overall high level of satisfaction, but patients saw room for improvement in information provided before and after medical examinations.[21]

Focus group participants wanted a range of independent information on health and the financial aspects of health services: '*Health information should not only come from doctors, but also from political institutions. They should inform us about ongoing modifications and co-payments, when they are being introduced, how much and why'*.

Younger participants, in particular, stressed the point that the government and health organizations should take responsibility for improving access to information. They could foresee a time when health information was freely available via computer terminals in hospitals and health insurance offices, and they called for the establishment of health information centres in all regions.

Participants felt well informed about the fact that they could have a say in diagnostic and therapeutic decisions. They also felt well informed about general aspects of health and illness and knew enough about the prevention of diseases. Participants felt less well informed about the quality of hospitals and ambulatory care, and about independent contact points for patients in hospitals – for example, ombudspersons or patient counsellors. They wanted more access to information about the quality of GPs, specialists and hospitals and about the specialist interests and knowledge of doctors. The magazine *Focus*, which publishes evaluations of hospitals and doctors, was mentioned as an example of the way forward.

Information sources

Within the context of a study of health information on the internet, participants were asked about the health information sources they used. Doctors were the most popular source (31 per cent), followed by brochures (21 per cent) and the internet (18 per cent).[22] Women use advice published in print media more frequently than men. In spite of the wide diversity of information services, the doctor's assistance in interpretation is highly valued. In particular, older people turn to their doctor with questions on health – more than 75 per cent of the over-55s reported seeking medical advice, while one third of those in this age group obtained their information via the pharmacist and/or magazines.

A large range of printed materials for patients is produced and disseminated by different providers. The degree of professionalism in presentation and content varies. Some institutions produce their own brochures, while others are produced by the pharmaceutical industry. For example, 94 per cent of information magazines handed out by GPs in Berlin came from the pharmaceutical industry, and of the material that was available in waiting rooms, 84 per cent came from pharmaceutical companies.[23] Only a few of the brochures came from independent public welfare organizations or health insurance agencies.

Group members were asked which information sources they *trust* most. They placed most trust in their GPs (29 per cent) and their specialists (29 per cent): *'I can ask my doctor and he will tell me exactly what's the matter and what the different treatment possibilities are'.*

Next on the confidence scale were books, which were most trusted by 17 per cent. There were differences between younger and older people. The younger ones said that for information on symptoms they seek information via the internet or other public media before they consult their GP or a specialist: *'If I find any symptoms myself, I get scared. What could it be? Is it something bad? First I investigate, for example the internet, search for specific illnesses, compare symptoms, could it be that? Or that? Then I go to the doctor'.*

The least trusted information source was the pharmaceutical industry. Confidence in magazines and newspapers was also low. People often complained about the long and incomprehensible instructions for using medicines.

Health websites

The internet has become an important resource for both providers and users of health information. More than 24 million Germans (aged 14 to 69) are internet users, of whom 58 per cent are men, and 27 per cent of users are online on a daily basis.[24] In a German online survey, 38 per cent of those polled stated that they used health information on the internet at least once a month.[25] The proportion of female users is increasing across all age groups and the number of senior citizens who are discovering the web has risen by a factor of more than five during the last five years. Around 14 per cent of internet users are now more than 50 years old.[26]

The internet is increasingly proving to be an organ of information for and about self-help in health-related matters. Half of the federal associations and umbrella organizations for self-help are present on the internet and this number is still increasing. Around 50,000 users accessed these websites in 1999, compared to 17,500 traditional written or telephone requests during the same period.[27] Of the focus group members in our study, 50 per cent had access to the internet. They knew the internet as a source for health information and used it in addition to other information sources. One male participant said: *'Usually you only have ten minutes with the doctor, and then I simply use the internet and search for the information myself'*. Around 15 per cent of users have changed their attitudes to the subject of health or to the doctors treating them as a result of information obtained on the internet.

The possibility of obtaining information from other countries was considered especially attractive: *'And there you are somewhere near Munich with the possibility of getting good information worldwide. Without the internet you would never find this kind of information'*. But participants saw difficulties in the abundance and variety of information on the internet: *'I feel that the internet overwhelms me and gives me more information than in fact I need'*. Furthermore it is difficult to find high-quality health information: *'There are fabulous websites in the case of certain illnesses with lots of information, but on balance you only find rubbish'*.

Participants criticized websites on the one hand for being too superficial and lacking new information and on the other for being so complicated that a lay person cannot understand them. It was also felt that it is often unclear who is responsible for the websites.

The sale or supply of medicines and medical aids over the internet has already started. The internet has become, according to Glaeske, an open 'pill channel',[28] and medication not yet available in Germany or only available on prescription can be obtained this way. A particularly controversial example of this is the online sale of the potency aid Viagra.[29] Regulation of this market is still difficult and complaints or claims for compensation are virtually impossible. While some German pharmaceutical companies want this area clarified in law, most German health insurance agencies welcome the potential savings to be achieved through mail order medication via the internet.[30]

PATIENT EMPOWERMENT

Self-diagnosis, self-medication, self-care

Of all Germans, 90 per cent consult doctors at least once a year,[31] but a large number of less serious health problems are treated by people themselves. For example, 80 per cent of those polled in a study conducted by an association of drug manufacturers stated that they could treat a whole range of symptoms and illnesses themselves without going to the doctor.[32] In doing this, around 80 per cent feel quite confident in assessing when they should consult a doctor and when they can treat themselves. About 50 per cent of those surveyed considered it important that over-the-counter medicines are available which enable self-treatment in the case of minor complaints. The use of over-the-counter medicines has increased in the last ten years. Germans spent DM678 million in 1999 on vitamin preparations and this market has increased by 7 per cent since 1998.[33] Self-medication is also becoming an increasingly significant segment of the pharmaceutical industry (now over 1000 products). Of the 1.6 billion medication packs, almost half are for self-medication.[28] The increasing health-consciousness of the population is regarded as a guarantee of an increasing market.[34]

Focus group participants thought they had a responsibility to inform themselves: *'It struck me that one must inform oneself, that one cannot rely on the doctor to give all possible information and all the possible alternatives with any medical treatment'*. For those who are chronically ill, taking responsibility means *'Avoiding medicines which are not necessary . . . I can achieve something with medicines, but I can also achieve a lot through my own initiatives'*. Taking responsibility was seen as including aspects of compliance. Male participants specifically mentioned this: *'If I have a broken arm it is up to me to protect it and to influence the healing process according to the recommendations of the doctor, and not play – I exaggerate now – soccer with a broken arm'.* For younger participants, responsibility meant *'Informing themselves about risks, i.e. risky sports or smoking'* and the adoption of a healthy lifestyle.

In Germany there are more than 70,000 self-help groups, of which a large number are active in the health field. Social security law requires health insurance agencies to provide financial support for these groups. Self-help contact points (around 250 in Germany) are professional advice facilities sponsored by local authorities or charitable associations. They offer information and advice on self-help, support the setting up of groups and strengthen cooperation between self-help groups and professionals. For example, the Kassenärztliche Vereinigung Nordrhein set up a cooperation advice centre for self-help groups and doctors (KOSA). On request, this organization passes information on self-help groups to doctors and supports them in the referral of patients to these groups, as well as advising doctors and self-help groups on the possibilities of co-operation.[35] The public welcomes this type of support for self-help organizations, and 74 per cent describe the financial assistance given by the health insurance agencies as desirable.[2]

Focus group participants felt that self-help groups provide both theoretical knowledge and practical experience of chronic illness. They offer clear and comprehensive information via personal counselling or doctor-patient seminars. Doctors also use them as supplementary information sources. This is a sign of the increasing acceptance of such groups, but some members of the focus groups were critical of this trend: *'I feel that's like a cop-out. The doctors make it really easy for themselves. So you go to the self-help group and then you get the information'.*

According to some participants, self-help groups have a broader and deeper knowledge of their illness than a doctor. It was emphasized that patient groups not only offer information and support related to the disease, but also support the daily life of group members.

Involvement in treatment decisions

The idea of shared decision making is accepted in Germany, even though its implementation is dependent upon various factors. For older patients and patients with a low level of education, active involvement in decision making appears to be less relevant than it is for younger people and people from higher social classes.[36] The need for information and active participation is also dependent upon a person's state of health. The more serious the illness, the less people want to make autonomous decisions.[37] For some German patients, autonomy only means being able to ask questions, while for others it means actively making decisions.[38] The need to be treated as a human being and not as a number was considered 'very important' by 89 per cent of patients in outpatient care, while being taken seriously by the doctor was 'very important' for 90 per cent. In contrast, the wish to be considered as an equal partner in the treatment process was rated as 'very important' by only 43 per cent of those surveyed. Older people mentioned this less often than younger people, but there was no difference between acute and chronically sick patients or between men and women.[39]

Patients are frequently reserved and do not wish to burden the doctor with their questions, but focus group participants thought it was important to ask more questions and make more demands: *'I used to be so naive and did whatever the doctor said. Today I would say I scrutinize that'.* All the participants agreed with this more critical attitude towards health care. However, they felt it required a lot of commitment: *'And therefore you must have the kind of disposition to say, "I won't consider that". Then you read, you inform yourself'.*

Patients frequently felt that professionals did not support them in this critical approach and all participants were aware of situations in which this kind of self-assertion is not worthwhile. Someone who is seriously ill might not have the strength or the inclination to be actively involved in decisions about diagnostic procedures and treatments. Then you have to *'. . . rely on the doctor, before one feels able to talk about all aspects of the illness'.*

But old notions of paternalism are still prevalent. Even participants from self-help groups who might be presumed to take an active and questioning attitude towards their own health care considered that *'The doctor decides, and then one does what he says . . . then one gives in somehow'.*

Finally the question remains of who patients should trust and whose judgement they should accept. The following example from a female group participant illustrates the dilemma:

My husband has had TB and the children and I were examined regularly. The children were infected, but not sick. The paediatrician thought they should take antibiotics for six months just in case. Then we asked our GP who said that antibiotics would not be absolutely necessary and we should consider very carefully the pros and cons of this. Then we consulted another doctor. He recommended that we wait and see whether the children fell ill or not. Most people don't fall ill even if they are infected. Now I had to decide which doctor to believe.

Ultimately, patients are left alone in this situation and they need competent support.

Electronic patient-held records

All participants saw the relevance of an electronic medical record and were open to this idea. Repeat investigations could be reduced, leading to cost savings, and as the medical history would be recorded chronologically, physicians would have easy access to all data for an individual patient: *'If the doctor wanted to prescribe some medicine, he would be able to see from the card whether it was suitable for me or not'.*

One important issue was data protection. Some participants were concerned that their medical data could be provided to sickness funds or employers, particularly if people have had mental disorders: *'There I have objections – information could be passed on to the employer, for example. That could be abused'.* All focus groups mentioned this problem. They discussed ways of restricting access to the information through fingerprints or special code words.

Choosing where to receive care

In general, patients prefer care that is close to home and if possible on an outpatient basis, but half the insured population of Germany welcomes the possibility of being able to travel elsewhere in Europe to seek health care, particularly young people.[40] However, 31 per cent of those polled expressed the fear that care in Germany would become poorer within a pan-European system. Whether the willingness in principle to consult a doctor outside Germany actually results in consultation of international doctors has not yet been examined systematically, but there are individual reports from areas close to the border of German patients visiting dentists in Poland and Hungary.

In order to be able to make a choice between health care providers, people need information about their quality. Up-to-date published details on the quality of inpatient facilities arouse a high level of interest among consumers.[41,42,43,44] They want comprehensible, readily available information on the performance of health facilities, accessible via different media. However, these data are not available at the present time. The *Regional Health Ministers' Conference* has addressed patient needs and together with other organizations, including self-help groups, has agreed 'Goals for a uniform quality strategy in the health care system'. This agreement specifies that all health facilities should provide annual quality reports by the year 2003 and publish these in appropriate form.[45]

Focus group participants considered it important that the information was objective and subject to strict quality controls. Independent institutions should provide and monitor the data: *'Every doctor will say: I am the best and every hospital as well. But if you're concerned you ask the consumer headquarters: which doctor is really good? Or which hospital should I choose for my particular illness?'*

Greater transparency was seen as a way of improving quality management and encouraging a more consumer-oriented approach: *'In the wake of publication ... where the figures are good, the hospital will get more patients, where they are bad, they'll get fewer. Then the bad hospitals will see the situation and – hopefully – change things'.*

Some female participants felt it was possible to measure the quality of medical services by looking at the number of therapeutic or diagnostic procedures performed – for example, the number of mammograms per month or heart transplantations per year. One woman gave an example in the rehabilitation area: *'There is a register of several clinics for rehabilitation and if it says three patients with colitis and two with Crohn's disease per annum, then I already know that the doctors are probably not the experts for this disease. If I see another clinic listed where they have 120 patients per annum, then I know that this clinic has lots of experience'.*

Information about how often medical personnel in different institutions are trained and what kind of vocational training they have was also felt to be useful. The competitive element was also recognized: *'And the doctor is then forced to undergo further training in order to keep his/her patients'.*

Nevertheless, participants thought it unlikely that doctors and hospitals would voluntarily subject themselves to quality control measures and publicize the results: *'Transparency is reasonable in theory, but I don't believe it's possible in practice'.*

It was unclear to most participants how access to this information could be arranged. Health centres or agencies for consumer protection were suggested as providers of the information, as well as national or local statutory agencies.

NEW ROLES FOR THE CITIZEN

Strengthening patients' rights

Individual patients' rights are defined in various laws. There are the basic human rights (the right to life and physical integrity and the right to autonomy and self-determination), while the more specific situation relating to health care is regulated in the *Sozialgesetzbuch* (SGB – *Social Security Code*). In 1999, various representatives of patients' interests came together under the leadership of the Regional Health Ministers' Conference and a 'Charter of Patients' Rights' was drawn up. The patients' charter is being carefully monitored at present to see whether further measures should be adopted.[46]

Although the patient has extensive rights in theory, in practice equal and independent representation in the implementation of patients' rights has still to be realized. Many users of the health care system are not aware of their rights or find no support when trying to exercise them.[2,47] No less than 25 per cent of those polled in a population study felt that data protection was not given sufficient priority within the health field.

More than half of all focus group participants said they felt 'rather poorly' informed about their rights: *'We were amazed when we were asked about our rights here. One does not know them as a patient'*. But in the process of discussion it became clear that the participants actually knew a lot of their rights, but did not recognize these as rights, rather as general preconditions of health care or as general civil laws. The freedom to choose a doctor was referred to as a legal right by almost all groups. On the other hand, the right to complain or the right to make informed decisions was mentioned in only one group. The right to confidentiality in the doctor-patient relationship was not mentioned at all.

Patients felt their rights were not really guaranteed. They were particularly concerned about the extent of the doctor's liability: *'A dentist hurt me once quite badly, and I did not think that this was necessary. In fact I should have had compensation for personal suffering, however, who am I supposed to turn to in this case? Or if I go to the doctor and he gives me an incorrect diagnosis and I am given the wrong treatment, what shall I do then?'*

Some group members knew it was possible to contact the arbitration board of the doctors' chambers when they suspected a medical error or to speak to their health insurer. However, confidence in these arbitration boards was not very high: *'they look after their own'.* Many participants felt patients should have more influence on the arbitration boards.

There is a difficult balance between medical ethics and patient autonomy in the context of patients' rights. This was illustrated in one focus group by the problem of living wills:

We have now an example in the family. My grandma does not want any life-prolonging treatment of whatever kind. She wrote that down many years ago and that was legally binding. But the doctor said that he does not acknowledge this patient's wishes because his oath obliges him to save lives and to help every patient, regardless of these documents.

Participation in policy making

At present most German citizens have only an indirect influence on health policy decisions through the exercise of their right to vote. Although the views of patient associations are heard in parliament, these views usually carry less weight than, for example, the statements made by the representatives of the sickness funds or the employers who almost unanimously support stricter cost controls.

One area in which public participation is practised in Germany is at the regional health conferences.[48] Individuals and patients' representatives are invited to health conferences in order, for example, to jointly advance health promotion activities, to discuss questions of health care on a local level and where necessary to provide recommendations. These are then implemented subject to the commitment of the participants.[49] But the legal basis for public participation is not considered sufficient at the moment.[50]

In the *Konzertierte Aktion im Gesundheitswesen* (Concerted Action on Health Care), in which proposals for improving performance, efficiency and economy are coordinated, the Federal Ministry for Health also involves members from disability and consumer associations. The question of who can act as user groups' representatives on decision making committees has not been conclusively clarified.

Public involvement in policy making was important to focus group participants: *'For me the most important issue would be participation. And indeed I think it is also important that patients are represented in health insurance and on the federal committee for doctors'*. Participants estimated the influence of patients on health policy making as 'rather small' or 'small': *'And I mean, if we have the right to participate in policy making, we can say we don't want overworked doctors. Then we can put more pressure on hospital managers to hire more doctors'*.

When asked who should act as patient representatives on the various committees, self-help groups, family members and consumer groups were all mentioned. Politicians were not trusted to represent patients' interests. Participants felt the main precondition for becoming involved was the ability to genuinely influence decisions: *'I think if it is limited to people rubber-stamping the decisions the management or politicians have already made, that's no good'*.

FOCUS GROUPS

Seven focus groups were held between August and October 2001, details of which are shown in Table 3.1.

Table 3.1 The focus groups in the German study

Group	No. of participants	Age	Sex	Location	Health status
1	9	33–62	Female	Hanover	Chronic illness/ healthy
2	8	22–60	Male	Hanover	Chronic illness/ healthy
3	8	34–74	Female	Munich	Chronic illness
4	10	20–30	Male/female	Hanover	Chronic illness/ healthy
5	10	44–66	Male/female	Berlin	Chronic illness
6	7	32–42	Male/female	Hanover	Chronic illness/ healthy
7	7	34–65	Male/female	Celle	Chronic illness

NOTES

1 Wasem, J. (2000) Der Patient im Mittelpunkt, *Bdvb-special Gesundheits-ökonomie*, 2(10): 5–7.
2 Wasem, J. (1999) *Das Gesundheitswesen in Deutschland: Einstellungen und Erwartungen der Bevölkerung. Wissenschaftliche Analyse und Bewertung einer repräsentativen Bevölkerungsstudie*. Neuss: Janssen-Cilag Gmbh.
3 Föste, W. and Janßen, P. (1997) Finanzierungs und belastungsgrenzen des Sozialstaats im Urteil der Bevölkerung, in H.P. Haarland and H.J. Niessen (eds) *Schriftenreihe für Ordnungspolitik*. Köln: FiO Forschungsinstitut für Ordnungspolitik.
4 Polis, G.K.V. (2000) *Einstellung der Bevölkerung in Nordrhein-Westfalen*. München: Bergisch Gladbach.
5 Stegers, C.M. (1997) Deutschland: Patientenrechte, in C. Kranich and J. Böcken (eds) *Patientenrechte und Patientenunterstützung in Europa: Anregungen und Ideen für Deutschland*, pp. 78–88. Baden-Baden: Nomos Verlagsgesellschaft.
6 WHO-Europe (2000) *Health For All Statistical Database 1999*, http://www.who.dk/country/country.htm.
7 Mossialos, E. (1997) Citizens' views on healthcare systems in the 15 member states of the European Union, *Health Economics*, 6(2): 109–16.
8 Zentralinstitut für die kassenärztliche Versorgung in der Bundesrepublik Deutschland (2000) *Gesundheitszustand und ambulante medizinische Versorgung der Bevölkerung in Deutschland im Ost-West-Vergleich*. Köln: Deutscher Ärzteverlag.
9 SEKIS (2000) Nutzeranliegen an Patienteninformationen. Diskussionspapier zur Tagung. Bedarf und Qualität von Patienteninformationssystem aus Nutzersicht. Fachtagung zum Thema Patienten – Versicherte – Verbraucher. Berlin, 9 März.
10 Klingenberg, A., Bahrs, O. and Szecsenyi, J. (1999) Wie beurteilen Patienten Hausärzte und ihre Praxen? Deutsche Ergebnisse der europäischen Studie zur Bewertung hausärztlicher Versorgung durch Patienten (EUROPEP), *Z ärztl Fortbild Qual sich*, 93(6): 437–45.
11 Schwartz, F.W. (2000) *Die Qualität des deutschen Gesundheitswesens: Welche Potentiale haben die Reformansätze zu Struktur, Qualitätsmanagement und Vergütung?* Nürnberg: Vortragsmanuskript.
12 Braun, B. (2001) *Ablehnungen von Leistungen als Folge von Budgetierung sagen an den Wurzeln des sozialen Gesundheitssystems. Zusammenfassung der Ergebnisse einer Versichertenbefragung*. GEK Studien, http://www.gek.de.
13 Gesundheitsberichterstattung des Bundes (2001) http://www.GBE-bund.de.
14 Richter-Hebel, F. (1999) Warum kommen Patienten nicht wieder? Eine Praxis-Untersuchung, *Z Allg Med*, 75: 389–92.
15 *Verbraucher-Newsletter*, März 2001, http://www.verbrauchernews.de/verbraucher/abo.

16 Montgomery, F.U. (2001) Telematik im Gesundheitswesen: Mächtiges Potenzial für mehr Qualität, *KrV*, 53: 92–4.

17 Bundesverband der Arzneimittelhersteller (1997) Der Arzneimittelmarkt in Deutschland in Zahlen, http://www.bah-bonn.de/forum/download/index.html.

18 Kahrs, M., Marstedt, G., Niedermeier, R. and Schultz, T. (2000) Alternative Medizin – Paradigma für veränderte Patienten-Ansprüche und die Erosion medizinischer Versorgungsstrukturen? *Arbeit und Sozialpolitik*, 54(1/2): 20–31.

19 Gals, E. (2001) Nutzen und Praktikabilität genetischer Screening-programme in der GKV am Beispiel der Erbskrankheit Hämochromatose, *Arbeit und Sozialpolitik*, 3–4(55): 46–8.

20 Dierks, M. Personal communication.

21 Kassenärztliche Vereinigung Berlin (2000) Die Ergebnisse der Patienten-befragung und der Befragung der Ärzte liegen vor. Ärzte sind wichtigste Verfechter von Patienteninteressen Pressemitteilung der KV Berlin, http://www.kvberlin.de.

22 Wasem, J. and Güther, B. (1998) *Das Gesundheitssystem in Deutschland: Einstellungen und Erwartungen der Bevölkerung. Delphi. Studienreihe zur Zukunft des Gesundheitswesens.* Neuss: Janssen-Cilag Gmbh.

23 Linden, M., Gothe, H. and Ryser, M. (1999) Information the family physician gives his patients to take home: utilization, contents and origin of printed information, *MMW Fortschr Med*, 141(47): 30–3.

24 GfK Online-Monitor (2001) Ergebnisse der 7: Untersuchungswelle, http://194.175.173.244/gfk/gfk_studien.

25 ComCult (2000) Besuch von Online-Angeboten, http://www.comcult.de/ccstudie/onbesuch.htm.

26 W&V online (2001) Senioren im Internet, www.wuv-studien.de/wuv/studien.

27 Thiel, W. (2000) Kommunizieren ohne Angesicht: Chancen und Risiken des internets für die Selbsthilfe, in *Deutsche Arbeitsgemeinschaft Selbsthilfegruppen e.V. Selbsthilfegruppenjahrbuch 2000*, pp. 113–21. Gießen: Selbstverlag.

28 Glaeske, G. (2001) Gegen die Pillengläubigkeit hilft nur ein Aufstand der Experten, *Psychologie heute*, April: 52–8.

29 Eysenbach, G. (1999) Online prescribing of sildanefil (Viagra®) on the world wide web, *Journal of Medical internet Research*, 1(2): e10.

30 Kaesbach W. (2001) *Arznei aus dem Internet, Finanztest*, 2: 83.

31 Statistisches Bundesamt (2001) Daten zur Gesundheit der Bevölkerung, http://www.statistik-bune.de.

32 Bundesverband der Arzneimittelhersteller (1995) Der Arzneimittelmarkt in Deutschland in Zahlen, http://www.bah-bonn.de/forum/download/index.html.

33 Bundesverband der Arzneimittelhersteller (2000) Der Arzneimittelmarkt in Deutschland in Zahlen, http://www.bah-bonn.de/forum/download/index.html.

34 Radio Marketing Service, Branchenreport OTC.

35 KOSA (2001) Kooperationsberatung fur Selbsthilfegruppen und Arzte. Kassenarztliche Vereinigung Nordrhein, http://www.kvno.de.

36 Dierks, M.L., Bitzer, E.M., Lerch, M. *et al.* (2001) *Patientensouveränität. Der autonome Patient im Mittelpunkt.* Stuttgart: Akademie für Technikfolgenabschätzung in Baden-Württemberg (im Druck).

37 Rothenbacher, D., Lutz M.P and Porzsolt, F. (1997) Treatment decisions in palliative cancer care: patients' preferences for involvement and doctors' knowledge about it, *European Journal of Cancer*, 33(8): 1184–9.

38 Altmann, B. and Munch, K. (1997) *Meinen Korper kenne ich selbst am besten. Eine Studie zur Selbstbestimmung in Pflegesituationen aus Sicht von Patienten.* Berlin: Diplomarbeit an der Humboldt-Universitat zu Berlin, Medizinische Fakultat Charite, Institut fur Medizin-/ Pflegepadagogik und Pflegewissenschaft.

39 Dierks, M.L. and Bitzer, E.M. (1997) Patientenerwartungen und Patientenzufriedenheit. Unpublished report. Hannover

40 Zok, K. (1999) *Anforderungen an die Gesetzliche Krankenversicherung. Einschätzungen und Erwartungen aus Sicht der Versicherten.* Bonn: Wissenschaftliches Institut der AOK.

41 Test (1997) *Gute Besserung.* Berlin: Stiftung Warentest 11: 97–105.

42 Test (1999) *Hitliste der Hospitäler.* Berlin: Stiftung Warentest 11: 89–95

43 *Focus* (1997) Krankenhauser im Vergleich: 39–46.

44 DAK (Deutsche Angestellten Krankenkasse) (2000) Mehrheit fordert Datentransparenz im Gesundheitswesen. Ergebnisse einer Forsa-Studie. DAK Pressemitteilung [22.3.2000]

45 Gesundheitsministerkonferenz (1999) Ziele für eine einheitliche Qualitätsstrategie im Gesundheitswesen. Beschluss der 72. Gesundheitsministerkonferenz am 9./10. Juni 1999 in Trier, http://www.gqmg.de.

46 SVR – Sachverständigenrat für die konzertierte Aktion im Gesundheitswesen. (2001) Bedarfsgerechtigkeit und Wirtschaftlichkeit. Bd. 1 Zielbildung, Prävention, Nutzerorientierung und Partizipation. Baden-Baden: Nomos

47 Brunner, A., Wildner, M., Fischer, R. *et al.* (2000) Patientenrechte in vier deutschsprachigen europäischen Regionen, *Z f Gesundheitswiss*, 8(3): 273–86.

48 Brandenburg, A. von Ferber, Ch., Renner, A. and Winkler, K. (1999) Gesundheitskonferenzen als kommunaler Handlungsprozeß, in *Public-Health-Forschungsverbünde in der Deutschen Gesellschaft für Public Health e.V.* (Hrsg.) (*Public-Health-Forschung in Deutschland*), pp. 245–53. Bern: Hans Huber.

49 Wismar (2001) Personal communication.

50 Hart, D. (1999) Bürgerbeteiligung im Gesundheitswesen: Rechtliche Analyse und Perspektiven, *Public Health Forum*, 7(26): 7–9.

4

ITALY

OPINIONS ABOUT THE HEALTH CARE SYSTEM

The present system

Italy's health system is a mixed, predominantly public one. There is a national public service (the NHS), but the private sector covers almost all areas of medical care, from general practice to specialist and hospital medicine and paramedical activities. The health service is still considered national in Italy, not merely by convention but because health care policy and management depend more on central than regional or local government. Even so, the NHS will in all likelihood be the most significant test of federalist reform. Decentralization now appears both inevitable and imminent.

The Italian health service appears to be marked by inequalities in the delivery of health services around the country, with notable spending and contributory differences among the regions. Generally, welfare spending favours the more developed regions of the centre-north. It follows that a more flexible organization of public powers must aim to redress this imbalance.

Access and responsiveness

According to European Commission figures, Italy's national health system scores the lowest satisfaction rating in the EU.[1] More than half the population (59 per cent) declare themselves very or quite dissatisfied with their health system and 33 per cent believe it needs to be completely overhauled. In a 1996 survey of 10,000 individuals of all social classes throughout the country, the health service achieved the worst ratings in a list of public services: 69 per cent of respondents deemed it unsatisfactory, rating it worse than unemployment agencies, tax offices, public transport and social security.[2] However, the views of people who had had recent contact with the Italian NHS (i.e. in the six months prior to the survey) were more positive, with 62 per cent declaring themselves satisfied.

Focus group participants, particularly those living in the centre-north, mentioned some positive and rewarding experiences featuring competent medical staff, a willingness to look for solutions and efficient diagnostic equipment, as well as negative views: *'When they realized I had a serious problem, I saw doctors and organizations functioning well. In short, once they were able to understand the problem everything moved quickly'.*

Greatest dissatisfaction centred on the bureaucracy of the system.[3] Professionals were seen as overworked and underpaid, often suffering 'burn-out' which negatively affects their professional performance and reduces the efficacy of the caring relationship:

I had to go to some offices, go through crazy procedures, jump from one office to the other without getting anything done.

In hospitals there aren't any sheets and pillows and we have to bring them from home. It was very dirty under the bed, and the nurse told me that if I didn't like it I could get a broom and clean it myself.

There was a clear distinction between perceptions and experience. When personal experience is positive the NHS appears to be 'the ideal treatment place'; on the other hand, when it is negative the whole NHS becomes a malfunctioning body in which problems are only solved by luck.

Recent polls showed that most people had a high degree of confidence in centres for research, specialist medicine and general medicine, but confidence in public health institutions with administrative responsibility (i.e. the Health Ministry and Local Health Corporations) was much lower.[4,5] Satisfaction with primary care services appears to be higher. A 1998 survey confirmed the very good opinion expressed by the majority of Italians of the services of GPs (82 per cent) and local analysis laboratories (76 per cent), which contrasted with a more critical view of public hospitals. Despite this, in the event of serious illness, 50 per cent of Italians continue to believe public institutions are more reliable, compared to 34 per cent who prefer to use private health care.[6]

Because of long waits, gaining access to public health services is undoubtedly more difficult than accessing private services. This problem was reported by 43 per cent of Italians.[7] Access to the services of local health corporations entails a wait in the clinic in excess of 20 minutes for a large percentage of users.[8] These inconveniences are experienced more often by people in the south and the islands (45 per cent) than those in the north-east (26 per cent). It comes as no surprise therefore to discover that service users in these areas of the country have a less positive opinion of service opening hours.

The problem of long waiting times was echoed by focus group participants: *'Each time I have to be examined it takes all day. I stand for hours in the queue waiting for my number to be called. Yesterday I made an appointment for an MRI for my brother-in-law and he has to wait 90 days. For my heart problem I had a test in January and they called me for the surgery in September'.*

As a result, many Italians seek the help of intermediaries who can ensure a higher quality service and easier access. In 1987 more than 39 per cent of people surveyed said that they had turned to someone – a friend or a hospital doctor – for help when seeking access to health services.[9] This proportion had declined by 1998 when only 22 per cent resorted to this strategy, possibly a sign of a perceived improvement in access to and reliability of health services.[6]

Many focus group participants (particularly from the south) thought that 'personal recommendation' was the only way to get the best out of the NHS – to get accurate information and diagnoses, avoid waiting, make quick appointments and receive better treatment:

> *If you want to be helped in Italian hospitals you have to know a doctor or a friend otherwise you don't get anywhere. You have to stand in queues, wait, you are not examined well. When I took the electrocardiogram to the professor he told me he couldn't admit me and luckily at that moment a lady came out. She was the wife of a judge we knew, so the professor took me arm-in-arm and he had me immediately admitted.*

There was a general feeling that 'personal recommendation' was unfair but unavoidable.

Structure and organization

Generally Italians feel that central government still has the greatest ability to influence Italy's health system, even though its role will gradually diminish in the future. The influence of the regions, local authorities, local health corporations, citizen and consumer protection organizations, associations representing the sick and private health organizations is seen to be very much on the rise. This picture was reflected in the 1992 'counter-reform', which redistributed power from central government to the regions and local health corporations, and expressly recognized the role of citizen representation (citizen and consumer protection organizations and associations representing the sick). Most focus group participants thought the NHS would undergo significant changes in the future from both a management and a clinical point of view, but they were convinced that these changes would make the system worse not better.

Most people (85 per cent) believe the NHS should continue to offer all types of service.[6] As far as Italians are concerned, growing recourse to the private sector (with spending in 1998 reaching 36 per cent of that in the public sector and 26 per cent of total spending) in no way implies a decline in the role of the public service. It is simply an expression of more choice within the framework of a broader range of services. Italians view the ability to choose between public or private health care in a positive light. Only 11 per cent of those surveyed thought it represented a wasteful duplication of resources.

Cost and efficiency

Since 1978 the NHS has offered compulsory health insurance coverage for the whole population. The main sources of NHS funding include regional taxation collected from businesses, general taxes and duties that flow into the National Health Fund, which is shared among the regions, as well as patient co-payments. Within this framework, the idea of paying an additional contribution for several services appeals to a sizeable minority of Italians: 27 per cent for Italy as a whole, rising to a third among younger people and university graduates.[5] In short, 'pay more to get more' is a logic that appeals most to those segments of the population that are more inclined towards social innovation, while older people and those with a lower level of education are much less willing to accept this option.

Ever since 1992, drug policies have been at the centre of plans to redefine the Italian NHS. In particular, efforts have been made to radically reform methods and criteria for the public funding of pharmaceuticals. The *Commissione Unica del Farmaco* reclassified medicines into three groups (therapeutic efficacy being equal): Category A, free; Category B, with 'co-payment, or prescription charge' – 50 per cent of sale price; Category C, to be met wholly by the patient. The 2001 finance law, abolishing prescription charges and the B category has completely overturned this situation.

Measures to control spending on medicines have been particularly intense and for three years (1993–5) there was a decline in public funding of pharmaceuticals. The opinions expressed by Italians on this point were particularly critical. Over 76 per cent of those interviewed felt there was insufficient funding for the purchase of medicines, with users having to pay for essential medicines out of their own pocket, while 24 per cent thought that funding was sufficient since really useful medicines are provided free of charge. People suffering from poor health tended to express negative judgements most frequently.[6]

Equity

Regional inequalities in access to health services have led to a significant number of patients seeking treatment in regions other than where they live. In 1998, for example, over 750,000 Italians travelled to other regions for routine hospitalizations for the treatment of acute illnesses and for rehabilitation treatment.[10] Regions in the north tended to import patients, while those in the south exported them. However, focus group participants pointed out that this option was not open to everyone: *'It is only for privileged people because you need money to move, it has to be a real necessity. If you don't have money you can't move, travelling is expensive'*.

All focus group participants had a strong belief that the Italian NHS would get closer to the American model, which they did not like because of prohibitive costs and in-built inequity: *'I am afraid it will become a system similar to the American one where each one pays for what he needs and this will be a loss because now we can use various treatments irrespective of how much money we have'*. They viewed with alarm the prospect of a two-tier system: a quality service for people with high incomes or a good insurance scheme, and a second rate service for those who cannot afford to pay. Feelings of uncertainty and worry prevailed among the middle/lower classes because it is these people who will suffer the consequences of any change in this direction: *'We can't all pay for insurance. The problem will be for the middle class because the lower class will have assistance anyway, but what will happen to the middle classes who can't pay for insurance?'*

Most focus group participants felt the NHS was qualitatively superior and more clinically advanced than private health organizations, because it carries out scientific research and the doctors deal with a larger and more varied caseload: *'I have a good opinion of the health service. In my opinion they have good equipment and good doctors. In public organizations they carry out research, they are connected with universities, they are more advanced'*. Only a few people, mainly from the south of the country, thought that private health care was better than public. These people had a strong belief that if you pay more for treatment you get better quality and a more caring attitude towards the patient: *'Since I pay they have more time for me'*.

PATIENTS' VIEWS OF HEALTH PROFESSIONALS

Doctors

Surveys conducted at national and local level in the 1980s identified the changing doctor-patient relationship as one of the most significant indicators of changing health-related behaviour. From those surveys the physician was judged not only by their medical knowledge but also by their ability to view the symptoms more holistically. In this sense the 'physician-psychologist' was much preferred to the 'physician-technician'. At the same time there emerged expectations of a more equal and transparent doctor-patient relationship. While more recent surveys confirmed these trends, they registered a slight but significant shift. With regard to the qualities characterizing a good doctor, people frequently mentioned professional capacity and experience (58 per cent).[6] If we add to this the 11 per cent who emphasized the importance of continuous study and training, it is clear that Italians place considerable emphasis on technical quality. Only 13 per cent of Italians perceived the ability to explain clearly to the patient the details of their illness as an important quality of a good doctor. A different, more cooperative and equal doctor-patient relationship, while being appreciated by Italian patients, is no substitute for medical expertise.

Most participants in the qualitative research felt they did not have enough power and control over their own clinical situation, because health professionals appeared distant and detached, not very willing to explain pathologies, treatments, length of hospital admissions or surgical options: *'The doctor treats the patient with cynicism, detachment and superiority: "I won't explain it because you won't understand". I think understanding what's being done is fundamental. The doctor always tells me not to worry but I have to know why'.*

However, patients demonstrated a degree of ambivalence. On the one hand they wanted more control and better information, the opportunity to take the lead in the therapeutic process, be better informed and have the right to choose. On the other hand, they were afraid of appearing arrogant and presumptuous, and questioning the doctor's competence and authority.

The family doctor's role was positively evaluated by participants who described their GP as a friend, a confidante, always available and ready to listen, a relationship that consolidates and deepens over time: *'I had a simple problem and I only saw the family doctor. He advised me to see a specialist but I only trusted him, he has known me for many years'.*

It was suggested to focus group members that they might reduce waiting time in the future by seeing a different doctor. Most participants reacted negatively to this proposal, because it would reduce the sense of a relationship with the doctor, jeopardize continuity of care and remove the patient's uniqueness and individuality: *'It isn't good to go one day to this one and the other to that one. It's better to be always treated by the same doctor because you establish a really human relationship. In my opinion the continuous relationship and therefore the knowledge of the patient's history is very important from a therapeutic point of view'.* Only a very few – all healthy young people – thought that this option would be useful in emergencies, when you really cannot wait for your own doctor, or when you want to exercise the right to choose in order to reduce waiting times: *'If one needs to be treated immediately it is OK. If my problem is urgent I go to the first doctor who is available. I think it's a decent choice option, as the patient likes, according to his needs'.*

Nurses

Nurses were seen as performing only support duties (e.g. the physical management of the patient, administering treatments, practical advice etc.) and focus group participants did not see a role for them in taking on direct responsibility for diagnosis and therapy: *'They are a support for the doctor. The nurse is not a substitute for the doctor. It is a matter of responsibility, nurses aren't competent'.* This negative perception of the nurse's role stemmed from the fact that paramedical personnel are considered inferior to doctors. There is still a hierarchy based on strictly defined roles. Therefore despite individual skills and/or experience acquired in the field, patients did not recognize any authority in nurses, whom they would never ask for suggestions or opinions on diagnoses or treatments.

Pharmacists

A recent survey set out to pinpoint the role that is implicitly attributed to pharmacists through an analysis of the type of information most frequently requested by their customers. The most common questions concerned instructions for taking purchased drugs (45 per cent). In the same category were requests for information on contra-indications and side-effects (43 per cent of questions).[11] People also wanted opinions on the effectiveness of medicines. In this case the pharmacist is clearly asked to offer a medical judgement, demonstrating a recognition of their specific knowledge and professional experience. People also wanted the pharmacist to tell them about compatibility with other medicines and with foods.

Most participants in the focus groups trusted pharmacists for advice on over-the-counter medicine or to solve minor indispositions but they did not foresee a widening of their role: *'Pharmacists know about over-the-counter products but they don't have the doctor's experience. There has to be a limit, they can't go further'.* This perception seems to originate from the fact that pharmacists no longer prepare medicines and have acquired an image closer to a shopkeeper.

ALTERNATIVE WAYS OF ACCESSING HEALTH ADVICE

Telephone

The possibility of conducting long-distance consultations through instruments such as the telephone and telemedicine foreshadows major developments in the near future. In a recent survey, 43 per cent of Italians expressed knowledge of telemedicine, while 67 per cent were aware of telephone helplines, thanks to TV campaigns. The majority of those interviewed believed these tools were very useful.[6]

The idea of using the telephone to consult a health professional provoked contrasting reactions among the focus group participants. People were keen on the idea of being able to consult various specialists (even in other parts of the world), but some had reservations:

'It's a good idea for people who have rare diseases, diseases for which they can't find a cure. It's useful when you find out that a specialist is in Germany and you can contact him to hear his opinion'.

Direct contact with the doctor was considered to be very important psychologically because it provides reassurance and comfort and helps to reduce anxiety: *'The doctor uses a stethoscope, touches, checks pressure. How do you do this on the phone?'*

Some participants felt it was unlikely that a telephone consultation service could be implemented because of costs and lack of availability of doctors: *'The doctor wouldn't answer the phone. He would pretend he isn't there. Just think if he is a chief physician he wouldn't talk to anyone. Here they only speak to who they want, to others they always tell their secretaries to say they aren't there'.*

Telemedicine

In general all participants thought that telemedicine was not likely to become a reality in the near future, but it provoked different reactions from men and women. Women were critical of the idea because it evoked coldness and detachment. Men and younger respondents were more enthusiastic. They were familiar with the technology and liked it, and understood the value of being able to consult professionals anywhere in the world, without limits or boundaries and at a convenient cost (the internet costs less than the telephone): *'Let's think how useful it is in important, serious cases, to get in touch with a famous specialist. We're talking about video link, so even if the person isn't physically there it is like they were'.*

EXTENDING THE SCOPE OF MEDICAL CARE

Complementary therapies

Results from a recent survey show that the number of people in Italy using the principal alternative therapies doubled between 1991 and 1999.[12] Despite this, Italy remains at the bottom of the relevant European league table. In 1999, 9 million Italians declared that they had used alternative treatments in the three years prior to the interview – 16 per cent of the population. The most common types of alternative therapies used were homeopathy, massage, herbal remedies and acupuncture. Alternative therapies were used by 5.5 million women and 3.5 million men. Of the interviewees, 40 per cent believed such treatment to be beneficial even though they did not have direct experience.

The degree of satisfaction is high among people who have tried these therapies: almost 70 per cent of those who have experienced different therapeutic approaches declared themselves to have benefited. The growing use of such therapies appears to be inspired by the belief that they are natural medicines and thus less harmful, but also by the positive evaluations given of practitioners who administer such treatment. They are perceived to be more sympathetic to patients' problems and deal with them on a more personal level.[6]

Participants in the recent focus group research reflected the generally limited acceptability of complementary medicine in Italy. It still seemed relatively unfamiliar and among the majority of respondents it provoked curiosity, scepticism and outright rejection: *'I am absolutely against it because I think anyone who uses these therapies is tied to an antique culture. Maybe they think they have the witch's potion that could be miraculous, more than the medicine the doctor prescribes'.*

Many patients' opinion of alternative medicine in general, and of homeopathy in particular, seemed to be influenced by the doctor. If they were against it, so was the patient. But everyone, irrespective of their personal opinion, felt there should be freedom to choose and that the NHS should recognize alternative medicine.

New medicines and biotechnologies

Italians do not necessarily see the unlimited expansion of health care services as a positive and desirable development. Focus group participants thought that the NHS should not concern itself with 'lifestyle' issues (e.g. treatments for baldness, impotence etc.) because they are not real illnesses and only represent needs induced by fashion and psychological problems: *'If someone has a crooked nose and has it straightened because they have breathing problems, that's one thing, but if they do it for aesthetic reasons, they should pay for it'.* One participant was in favour of the NHS providing this type of treatment, but only if the problem creates suffering and is threatening the patient's quality of life: *'A crooked nose, in my opinion, can become a disease because if that poor person looks at himself in the mirror every morning and suffers because he doesn't like himself, then he doesn't live well and it is right that the health system should help him if he can't afford to pay'.*

Data obtained from a survey conducted in 2001 show that

biotechnologies are no longer a mystery to Italians. Indeed they have high expectations of them. Of the interviewees, 62 per cent believed that biotech research might lead to the discovery of new therapies for treating diseases such as cancer or Alzheimer's, and more than 55 per cent of the sample expressed the belief that such research would make it possible to defeat genetic and other serious diseases.[5]

There was little concern about potential discrimination deriving from the improper use of genetic tests capable of predicting people's predisposition to particular diseases. All focus group participants were in favour of progress in the genetics field, but most of them would only undergo tests if they were prescribed by the doctor. Indeed these types of tests stimulated anxiety. Knowing about a predisposition to a serious disease made patients feel they were under 'sentence of death': '*You feel the sword of Damocles over your head. We have to be fatalistic in life. If I know I have a predisposition to a disease for which they haven't found a cure, well, why should I know about it, I'm going to wait and see*'.

INFORMATION FOR PATIENTS

Health information needs

Most Italians (77 per cent) say they want authoritative information to guide and help them with important health matters.[5] Of these, 63 per cent wanted detailed information, while 16 per cent would be happy with just the essential elements. Patients need help in finding their way through the large amount of information available.[5] Half of the respondents complained that it is very difficult to choose the right doctor or the right hospital because there is such a wide choice. An even greater number (63 per cent) reported difficulty in finding information about the increasing number of drugs now available.

The physician still plays a central role in providing information. GPs and television are, in that order, the preferred points of reference for Italians for this kind of information, but the role of the GP declines in importance as the patient's level of education rises.[6] While 83 per cent of those with no formal educational qualifications said GPs were their main source of information, the percentage fell to 46 per cent for more educated people, who also frequently consult specialist and popular publications and relatives, friends and colleagues.

A general picture emerges of people wanting to liberate themselves whenever possible from the traditional experts. Further confirmation of this tendency comes from the growing number of specialist publications such as medical encyclopaedias and books on medicine, natural medicine and psychology, and the proliferation of television programmes dealing with prevention and medicine. Apart from broadcasts dealing with topics relating to healthy living, diet and exercise, programmes focusing on specific health problems enjoy good viewing figures on the main public and private television channels.

Information sources

The focus group discussions demonstrated that information sources are used differently depending on whether the information is to satisfy a need or a curiosity. For the newly diagnosed patient, the most reliable and trustworthy sources were considered to be the family doctor, word of mouth and relatives/friends. In particular, respondents saw the doctor to get information, not only on the specific disease, but also on therapies, drugs and their possible side-effects, clinical tests and how to prepare for them. Information sought from friends and relatives mainly concerned specialist centres, waiting times, ways to access services and professional competence. The exchange of experiences was perceived as the most reassuring and efficient way to be informed: '*A friend of mine has had a high cholesterol level for five years and he knows what to do and where to go, so when the doctor diagnosed it I immediately asked him*'.

Most participants did not trust advice given in magazines and on television programmes because they thought they were not very credible, contradictory and in some cases even dangerous, too concerned with commercial interests and ratings, or dictated by the latest fashion trends: '*In the same magazine there was a page with the carrot diet, and some advice on following the carrot diet. Then there was an article written by a professor saying not to go on magazine diets because they are dangerous. How can we believe it?*'

Finally, only a very few were interested in brochures available in doctors' surgeries. Although they may contain advice and news on primary prevention or ways to manage a disease, people rarely keep them and usually only read them to kill time while waiting.

Health websites

In Italy, according to the *Italy Internet Observatory*, the number of 'surfers' rose from around 5 million in June 1999 (7 per cent of the population) to roughly 10 million at the end of the same year (about 18 per cent of the population). The number of health-related websites is growing rapidly. It is estimated that around 4 million Italians seek health-related information on the web. Moreover, 61 per cent of the Italian population is in favour of the possibility of having an online physician to answer questions. People appear to be aware of the enormous potential of the internet: 60 per cent of those interviewed saw it as a useful way of obtaining health-related information, with younger people and those with higher education being especially positive.[5]

Attitudes among the focus group participants varied. Younger people were enthusiastic and believed the internet could be useful for getting information on scientific research, finding out about new treatment methods, treatment centres, booking appointments etc. Men saw the internet as offering new possibilities that could improve communication between doctors, provide advice, generic information and news on drugs. Women were less enthusiastic, perhaps because they were less familiar with computers.

PATIENT EMPOWERMENT

Self-diagnosis, self-medication, self-care

Most focus group participants said they looked after themselves in the case of minor illnesses, like flu and colds. They had acquired the experience to do this over many years, they knew the correct medication for the problem and did not ask the doctor's advice, although they might discuss it with the chemist first.

Participants were convinced that prevention was important in order to keep healthy and avoid disease, but there were some differences of opinion. Women tended to go for regular check-ups to prevent female and dermatological cancer (e.g. breast cancer, cervical cancer, melanomas etc.). In contrast, most of the men said they did not give any priority to prevention programmes, they did not undergo recommended specialist screening and they only treated the diseases they knew they had: '*I would undergo prevention only if I knew there was a solution to a problem I was looking for. I prefer not knowing anything. I check only when I don't feel good. I don't stay there checking on what I could have'.*

Most patients with chronic diseases monitored their own health (especially those with hypertension or diabetes) and checked their blood pressure and sugar levels, using electronic gauges that can be purchased at the chemist. But some patients did not trust self-monitoring and liked to see the doctor to confirm their own results at home: *'Now with these electronic gauges it is enough to put them on and they do everything on their own, but I always go to the doctor, to receive confirmation'.*

In Italy, *self-care*, including therapies ranging from self-medication to the use of 'non-conventional' medicines and forms of non-medical self-treatment (rest, diet etc.), has not been the subject of systematic studies. Although it is not possible to make precise judgements about the spread of self-care practices among the population, an analysis of some indirect indicators and the results of some surveys reveal some interesting points.

In 1997, 33 per cent of the population had taken medicine of one sort or another in the two days prior to the survey, 28 per cent of men and 37 per cent of women.[13] But in the great majority of cases, medicines were prescribed by the doctor (in 87 per cent of cases, and 100 per cent for over-75s). Almost all interviewees said they usually check the expiry dates of medicines and read the warnings and instructions. Italians thus show a responsible attitude and are aware of the risks associated with the improper use of pharmaceutical products. This is borne out by another survey that found that 61 per cent of Italians believed that medicines should be used with considerable caution, under close medical surveillance and only in certain cases.[6] A significant percentage of the sample (41 per cent), believed the easy availability of medicines in modern society is excessive and difficult to keep up with.

Involvement in treatment decisions

The role of the physician is still secure and unquestioned in the eyes of Italians, and GPs in particular remain the point of reference for important health decisions. However, patients are beginning to claim their right to have a say in such matters. For the majority of those surveyed, decisions on medical treatment are seen as the responsibility of the patient, at least in part, for both serious and less serious illnesses. This view is the result of fairly recent cultural changes so it is not surprising that there were different views depending on the age and level of education of respondents. Among elderly and less educated people there is much less talk of an active role for the patient in the decision making process. More than 26 per cent of those over the age of 64 believe the patient should have no role in decisions about serious illnesses, compared to 17 per cent of those between the ages of 18 and 29, 25 per cent of persons only in possession of a junior school-leaving certificate and 13 per cent of graduates.[4] While only 10 per cent of interviewees agreed with the idea of the physician becoming a mere provider of information, 64 per cent of Italians favoured the idea of a cooperative type of relationship.

Electronic patient-held records

The proposal that everyone could carry their medical history on an electronic card was welcomed by most participants in the focus groups because it introduced a concrete solution to a deeply felt problem – that of personal records. Patients are often uncomfortable while giving a medical history because they are not familiar with medical language, and are afraid of forgetting information that could be important for the correct diagnosis. Participants liked the idea of the smart card, because it could be used anywhere, it could carry a lot of information and it would reduce the possibility of misdiagnosis, mixing up notes etc.: *'Once we have everything registered on a card we could access all information. We wouldn't need to worry about remembering everything . . . because if I am the one there explaining it's easy for the doctor to make a mistake'.* Only a few participants criticized the idea on the grounds that it could infringe rights to privacy and confidentiality. Some people were concerned that data could be altered or misdiagnoses inserted in the smart card.

Choosing where to receive care

The focus group participants initially found the idea of publishing indicators of the quality of care from different providers interesting because it offers patients a real opportunity to choose and could increase autonomy and a sense of responsibility: *'It's a good thing to have more information so one can choose who to go to. Furthermore you can find out if they are better in Liguria or in Florence and decide where to go'.* But some doubts emerged concerning the delivery and quality of information: *'Who will guarantee this information?*

Will it be a serious information network or maybe for a series of reasons they will prefer one doctor to another or one centre to another . . . I wouldn't trust this service'.

In particular, participants felt confused about the type of information that would be available. They wanted extremely detailed information about the safety, efficiency and technical quality of hospitals and specialist centres, and about the specialization and reliability of doctors and other health professionals: *'They also have to say that a certain doctor has treated two cases and both patients died while another one treated 200 and no one died. They have to provide a series of cases of what he did and the results he obtained'.* They felt there was also a risk that some hospitals or doctors would become overloaded because if they got good results everyone would want to be treated there. Certain information could lead to the creation of two classes of doctors: *'Top quality and poor quality doctors would emerge and this could be dangerous for their profession'.*

From the patients' point of view, there was felt to be a limit to how much information some people would be able to cope with. A lack of familiarity with medical terminology could make it difficult to make a decision and the patient might feel even more on their own. In fact some (particularly in the south) were convinced that it was the hospital's or doctor's duty to suggest and help the patient with choices and decisions: *'It depends on your knowledge of medicine. I can see that it would be difficult for many people to manage this information and keep control of their situation'.* So this idea created confusion and disorientation in participants since it conflicted with the need for reliability, support and security:

> *I don't think it's feasible. Who would say about himself don't come to this hospital because they are all dogs but go somewhere else because they are very good? Then we have to consider how objective the person is who gives the information, if he doesn't have any interest or doesn't earn anything when suggesting one doctor instead of another one.*

NEW ROLES FOR THE CITIZEN

Strengthening patients' rights

Article 32 of the Italian constitution safeguards patients' rights. Since the late 1970s, numerous organizations have been set up in Italy to defend the rights of the sick. These include voluntary welfare organizations such as the Tribunal for Patients' Rights and citizens' organizations that promote the notion of 'active citizenship'.

In 1980, Italy adopted the first charter for the rights of the sick, aimed at uncovering malpractice. Since then around 80 charters have been produced, and many of them have been incorporated into the regulations of local health corporations. Since 1997 the Tribunal and the Democratic Federation Movement have been working on the Integrated Plan for the Defence of Citizens' Health Rights (*PIT salute*). This operates as a database and monitors the relationship between citizens and the health system. In its first two years of activity the PIT registered 40–45,000 complaints. These mainly concerned access to, and quality of, services. Compared with the situation in 1997, there seems to have been a marked deterioration in access, particularly the acquisition of medicines, while the quality of services appears to have improved.[14]

The implementation of service charters is at an advanced stage, yet the reaction of the public has been disappointing. In 1998 just 22 per cent of those interviewed were aware of the existence of a health services charter, and although the majority of Italians believed it to be a useful tool, 34 per cent of the population was unable to form an opinion on the subject, revealing the persistent and widespread lack of information about such initiatives.[6]

The growing intolerance of medical errors is reflected in the amount of media attention given to such cases and in the increase in compensation claims and payments. During 2000 there were 143 cases of malpractice that resulted in more or less serious damage to patients, reported in 195 press articles. In many cases (55 per cent) the damage caused was fatal.[15] The 1990s saw a particularly marked increase in claims connected with health, from 10 per cent of total claims in 1991 to 15 per cent in 1999.[7] This bears witness to the public's growing awareness of their rights in relation to physicians and health organizations.

In the focus group discussions, participants thought the most important patient rights were the right to be treated (i.e. facilities for more disadvantaged areas, reduction of waiting times), the right to equal treatment (i.e. to receive the same treatment in public and private, no special treatment for those with the right contacts), the right to be treated with dignity (i.e. not being considered as a number, high standards of hygiene etc.) and the right to information (i.e. on disease, on treatments). Almost all participants stated that these basic rights were neither protected nor respected and they felt pessimistic about the possibility of any change.

Participation in policy making

After a long period when priority was given to increasing the availability of health services, recent financial difficulties have led to the idea of rationing or priority setting. In the Italian context, where the goal of ensuring uniform levels of health care for all citizens is hindered by powerful mechanisms of hidden rationing, attempts to tackle this problem may be seen as a means of bringing the issue out into the open and fixing transparent, fair and socially acceptable criteria. The debate is in its early stages, and is having some difficulties in finding its rightful place among proposals to revamp Italy's NHS.

A survey asked people to rank service priorities. Italians placed the treatment of seriously ill children at the top of the league table, followed by major surgery, such as organ transplants and operations in which patients' lives are at risk, mass vaccination to prevent disease, and special treatment and pain-killing therapy for the terminally ill.[16]

This list of priorities suggests a willingness to penalize specific groups, such as terminally ill over-75s and newborns with poor chances of survival (services for these groups come bottom of the table). But in general respondents rejected the idea of discrimination against specific user groups according to physiological characteristics (such as age) or unhealthy lifestyles (such as smoking, drinking etc.), while the quality of the future life of the patient is accepted as a parameter for determining whether life-saving treatment should be given or not.

Finally, when asked who should be given responsibility for rationing health spending, most Italians (39 per cent) indicated GPs, followed by the Health Ministry (20 per cent), local citizens' associations (16 per cent) and local health corporation managers (16 per cent). These results confirm the central role of the physician and the confidence placed in him by the public. The physician, being the repository of medical skills, is viewed as a guarantee against the risk of resource allocation based on anything other than effectiveness and appropriateness of treatment.

FOCUS GROUPS

Five focus groups took place in autumn 2001, details of which are shown in Table 4.1.

Table 4.1 The focus groups in the Italian study

Group	No. of participants	Age	Sex	Location	Health status
1	9	30–50	Female	Milan	Acute
2	9	50–65	Male	Florence	Chronic illness
3	9	18–30	Male/Female	Rome	Healthy
4	9	30–50	Male/Female	Bari	Acute
5	9	50–65	Female	Palermo	Chronic illness

NOTES

1 European Commission (1998) *Citizens and Health Systems: Main Results from a Eurobarometer Survey*. Brussels: Office for the Official Publications of the European Community.

2 Bosio, A.C. (1996) Report on the perceived quality of health services in Italy, in M. Trabucchi (ed.) *Citizens and the National Health System*. Bologna: Il Mulino.

3 Vecchio, C. (1997) Citizens – NHS – Physicians: relations to be updated, *Giornale Italiano di Cardiologia*, 27.

4 Censis Forum for Biomedical Research (2001) *New Patients and Biotechnologies*. Milan: Franco Angeli.

5 Censis Forum for Biomedical Research (2001) *Health-related Communication and Information*. Unpublished report.

6 Censis (1998) *Health Demand in the 1990s*. Milan: Franco Angeli.

7 Censis-Assomedico (2001) *Risks and Errors in Italian Health System*. Unpublished report.

8 Istat (2000) Health system and health of the population, *Informazioni*, 16.

9 Censis (1989) *Health Demand in Italy*. Milan: Franco Angeli.

10 Censis (2000) *34th Report on the Social State of the Nation*. Milan: Franco Angeli.

11 Censis (1997) *Medicines and Distribution*. Milan: Franco Angeli.

12 Istat (1999) *Health Conditions and use of Health Services 1999–2000*. Rome: Istat Publications.

13 Istat (1998) *Health Conditions and use of Health Services*. Rome: Istat Publications.

14 PIT (1998) *Citizens and Health Services. Report 1997–98*. Rome: PIT.

15 Censis analysis 2001.

16 Censis (1999) *Is it Right to Treat Everyone? Criteria for Health Rationing*, unpublished report.

5

POLAND

OPINIONS ABOUT THE HEALTH CARE SYSTEM

The present system

Under the totalitarian post-war Polish state of 1945–89, Poland's health service was controlled and financed by the state. Major political changes in the late 1980s led to reorganization of the health system and these changes have become the most important issue in the reform debate, overshadowing all others. In 1999 the old system was replaced by one financed through a health insurance scheme based on 17 independent regional sick funds and one fund that provides health care for the police and the military. The sick funds provide financial support to health care institutions under contracts that define productivity parameters. These contracts are confidential and even within the same sick fund the rates and limits for similar services vary widely.

The patient's status in contemporary Poland is influenced by history, athough changes are occurring aimed at improving the patient's position and adjusting the health services to patients' needs and expectations. The traditional, paternalistic system of health care is gradually evolving into one in which patients are given a greater choice of care providers. At the same time, however, access to health services has been reduced as a result of their partial privatization and the limitations introduced by the sick funds.

Access and responsiveness

According to surveys, seven out of ten Poles are dissatisfied with the functioning of the reformed health care service.[1] Concerns tend to focus on access and payment issues. The requirement to contribute co-payments means that some patients refrain from buying the medicines they need and seeing specialists and dentists, and postpone their hospital treatment, mainly for financial reasons.[2] Our qualitative research confirmed this dissatisfaction. Participants in the focus groups complained of costs, inefficiencies and excessive bureaucracy that also limits access to doctors, particularly specialists.

In evaluating the quality of health care, Polish patients place considerable emphasis on the qualifications of health professionals, the right to choose a doctor and the friendliness or otherwise of health professionals.[3] Other important factors include direct access to medical examinations and to specialists, and service efficiency, as well as high quality equipment, cleanliness and sterile care, and having a full range of services in one place.

The issue of access, and particularly access to GPs, is key. Research based on an all-Poland sample found that almost 50 per cent of respondents were discontented with this aspect of the system.[1] Some patients viewed limitations on access to specialists as another drawback of the reforms. The sick funds' requirement that referral to a specialist can only be made by a GP was unpopular with two thirds of respondents in one survey.[4]

People in the focus groups felt the lack of easy access to doctors was the weakest aspect of the national health service. They were of the opinion that high quality health services should enable quick access to specialists without referrals from GPs, especially to ophthalmologists, surgeons and laryngologists: *'There are specialists who have patients booked in three months ahead but for some people such a long wait may be a death sentence'*.

There was a strong belief among some participants, especially men, that high quality care can only be provided by specialists: *'A GP basically knows about a range of different illnesses but cannot treat specific dermatological and laryngological cases'*.

Some patients use informal channels to secure faster access to services. In a 1999 survey, 28 per cent said they were admitted to hospital after using one or more informal methods to secure admission. Informal channels include intervention by an acquaintance (a doctor or other health professional), private visits to hospital doctors and bribes. The predominant informal way of gaining admission to a hospital is still the intervention of a doctor friend.[5]

Structure and organization

A key component of the health service reforms begun in the early 1990s was the establishment of a GP or family doctor service responsible for basic medical care. GPs were expected to work in individual or group practices, and several thousand practices have started work in the last few years. GPs have contracts with the sick funds and exist alongside the remnants of the previous system: regional outpatient clinics with many specialists employed full-time. In cases requiring specialist treatment, a GP is expected to refer the patient to a specialist or to the hospital.

The new family doctor service has been well received by patients. In the first few months after the new system was introduced, nearly 38 per cent of patients registered with family doctors in the Lublin Province.[6] After one year, 52 per cent of respondents in this region were on GPs' lists. Patients expect a GP to provide comprehensive medical care for 24 hours a day, including home visits. They also want specialist tests to be done in the practice.[7] Parents, however, still indicate a preference for specialist paediatric care for their children.[6]

Cost and efficiency

Reform has meant that patients have to cover the cost of their health care to a greater extent than before. Certain services which were previously free of charge now have to be paid for. The cost of medicines has also increased significantly, partly because of opening the market to expensive imports and partly because of the deregulation of prices for generic medicines. Patients who cannot get the medical attention they need in the public sector or under health insurance coverage use private services. Focus group participants felt that private health centres provide better quality services than national health institutions and that private medical staff treat patients with more kindness: *'The truth is that we trust private health centres more than national ones because they provide better quality services and the patient is always welcomed there'*.

Obtaining medical care at their own expense in private health centres is not only a result of patients' conviction that these centres provide better quality services. It is just as likely to result from difficulties in accessing the required services through the health insurance system. During the period from July 1999 to January 2000, nearly 43 per cent of respondents to one survey reported using private services.[8]

The need to pay out-of-pocket for additional costs can have an adverse effect on health care utilization. One in three respondents (34 per cent) reported that they or one of their dependents had to give up treatment because of financial hardship in the six months from July 1999 to January 2000. Respondents most frequently refrained from buying prescription drugs or other pharmaceuticals recommended by a doctor (21 per cent); using dental services (14 per cent); or seeing a specialist (13 per cent).[9]

Attitudes to paying out-of-pocket for health care are related to educational level, social status and place of residence. The higher the level of education and social status of the respondents, the more willing they are to pay for medical services directly, rather than through an insurance system. Those living in big cities are more likely to favour individual payments while those living in the country prefer the insurance system.[8]

Equity

Most Polish people believe the government should be responsible for reducing inequalities in access to health care services.[10] This belief relates mainly to the financing of medical services and is less common among well educated or wealthy people who tend to feel that health care should be the responsibility of the individual. But they are the minority (about 7 per cent of Poles have university education and only 5 per cent pay the highest tax rate).[11] The majority (76 per cent) prefer to pay a compulsory insurance premium, and only 16 per cent opt for voluntary insurance (outside the official insurance system). Despite this, two fifths of Poles accept that they must contribute out-of-pocket payments to have decent health services.[8]

PATIENTS' VIEWS OF HEALTH PROFESSIONALS

Doctors

Patients' views on the health service depend mainly on their feelings about their physicians. Qualitative and quantitative research highlights the fact that patients consider doctors the most important individuals in the health care system. Trust in doctors remains high, with 63 per cent expressing high levels of confidence and 18 per cent saying they had complete confidence in their doctor.[12]

A fundamental characteristic that patients require in their doctors is empathy, an ability and willingness to acknowledge the feelings, reactions and circumstances of another human being.[13] The ability to empathize was highly valued regardless of the physician's specialization. Family doctors are expected to provide medical care and examine patients but also to offer moral support with social problems.[7] In other words, patients expect their GPs to act as psychologists and therapists.

Confidence in doctors may be judged by the frequency with which patients seek a second opinion. If it is low, the patient is more likely to consult another doctor. Patients who stress the importance of seeking a second opinion were less likely to express a lot of confidence in their doctor, but only 1 in 11 patients reported exercising this option.[12] Older people tended to show a higher degree of confidence than younger patients.

Within the focus groups, women and older men were rather reluctant to see another doctor if their 'own' doctor was not available, even if it meant a longer wait: *'Patients should definitely see their usual doctor as we know from our own experience that frequent change of doctors is not good and leads nowhere'*. Most patients seemed to trust their 'own' doctors more and were more convinced about the effectiveness of their treatment. Only in an emergency would they be prepared to see another available doctor: *'There are situations when we prefer to wait a fortnight for our "own" doctor, e.g. my gynaecologist because he has a very good reputation, rather than see another specialist who may be available but is an unknown quantity'*.

Focus group participants wanted health care to become more patient-centred and accessible. They wanted health professionals to show more kindness and doctors to have more time for patients. Group members were more concerned with human factors such as the doctor-patient relationship than with sophisticated medical equipment or high-tech medicine: *'The doctor-patient relationship should change first. Only then should other developments be used, like telemedicine'*. Most participants said they wanted professionals to listen to them, to empathize with them and respond to their emotional needs as well as their health problems.

There was general agreement among focus group participants that a good quality health service is based on sound working practices, a high level of competence among its medical professionals and a recognition of patients' needs. Most people tended to see themselves as customers with a right to high quality services, rather than as petitioner patients. Participants felt that GPs should be familiar with their past medical history so as not to refer them to specialists unnecessarily: *'Physicians are responsible for their patients and should not treat them in a slapdash manner as objects just wanting a prescription'*.

Participants felt that on some occasions the best role the doctor could play was to comfort the patient, give advice and recommend cheaper drugs in recognition of the patient's economic status. Group members thought that the more interested the doctor is, the quicker the recovery would be.

Focus group participants felt that doctors are often overburdened with bureaucratic responsibilities and do not have the time to establish good and satisfactory relationships with their patients. They mentioned situations when a hospital consultation started with filling in forms instead of providing emergency care. Writing notes can be so demanding and time-consuming that doctors lack the time to talk to their patients, who feel ignored: *'When a doctor deals with me hastily, because there are many waiting behind me, I feel neither satisfied nor safe'*. Some respondents suggested that doctors should have someone to help them with their clerical duties. They felt the health system must be blamed for the bureaucratic burden, not the doctors themselves.

Nurses

Generally, the nurse's role is highly valued by Polish patients. Studies indicate that the attributes considered most important are nurses' personal approach, friendliness, skill, efficiency and ready availability.[14] An individual, friendly approach to each patient is seen as producing confidence and reassurance, which has a positive effect on recovery.[15] Patients are more satisfied when given an opportunity to help plan their own treatment.[16] Thus a nurse is expected to not only assist the patient but also provide information on the progress they are making. When patients are denied such information they become insecure, which in turn negatively impacts on the therapeutic process.[17]

However, many focus group participants felt that the four-year training undertaken by nurses is not sufficient to qualify them for a more responsible role. Younger men, and those with only limited experience of contact with nurses, tended to downplay the role of the nurse, believing they are only qualified to carry out some of the less important tasks like assisting doctors or caring for the elderly and chronically ill. Older men with more experience of nursing care felt that nurses were overworked. They tended to feel that asking them to take on extra duties is not an example of professional autonomy but an attempt to burden nurses with responsibilities doctors do not want: '*Unfortunately nurses have a lot of work. I do not think they can do more. They often do work for doctors and lab staff and have no time to do anything else*'.

Women tended to believe that there were some situations where nurses (e.g. experienced, well-qualified midwives at natural child-births) should have more authority than doctors: '*The nurses often have the same level of professional knowledge as the physicians. However, they have to consult them about everything*'.

Participants felt that the burden on doctors could be reduced if nurses could legally prescribe what the doctor ordered. One group member reported that in some primary care health centres, nurses were already authorized to write repeat prescriptions for continuing treatments originally prescribed by a doctor. Several participants felt nurses should be entitled to prescribe certain medicines (e.g. analgesics, vitamins, diastolic drugs), provided there is some kind of supervision system to prevent errors.

Pharmacists

Generally, Polish patients have confidence in pharmacists and appreciate their role. They are perceived as partners of doctors in the process of medical treatment and as the number of over-the-counter medicines is now considerable (46 per cent of the pharmaceutical market), their advice on medication was seen as very important.[18] Features appreciated by patients are the pharmacist's readiness to help and their discretion. As with doctors, patients saw a clear connection between pharmacists' age and knowledge. They prefer an older person with considerable experience, thinking that such a person will have enough knowledge to suggest the correct remedy. Patients are against the proposal of abandoning doctor's prescriptions and leaving the choice of medicines in the hands of patients and pharmacists. They believe that the only person competent to prescribe is a doctor.[19]

In the focus groups, pharmacists' professional knowledge was valued more highly than nurses' when patients are seeking advice and information. Pharmacists can advise on over-the-counter medicines, give detailed information on drugs prescribed and recommend cheaper alternatives – an important consideration for many patients: '*The pharmacists have more knowledge than other medical professionals about medicines. They are able to advise when a patient wants specific information about a drug*'.

Older women in the focus groups felt that pharmacists should be able to prescribe analgesics and circulatory drugs if the patient's doctor had prescribed them before. Information about this service could be made available at the health centre reception. Some male participants believed that pharmacists are less exposed to the influence of pharmaceutical companies than doctors, making their choice of drugs more objective: '*Physicians often have a formal connection with the drug companies that makes them prescribe their medicines. The pharmacies tell us which medicines are cheaper and effective as well*'.

ALTERNATIVE WAYS OF ACCESSING HEALTH ADVICE

Telephone

Women in the focus groups were enthusiastic about the possibility of consulting health professionals over the telephone, especially if advice could be available on a 24-hour basis. A quick telephone consultation could save a lot of time and anxiety if parents were alarmed about symptoms in their children, or where advice was wanted on over-the-counter medicines. In cases where a specialist appointment was necessary, this could be obtained without queuing at a health centre. However, most participants felt that telephone consultations would only be appropriate for minor ailments. They thought that advice on more serious problems should be provided by a GP who knows the patient and their medical history.

Men were less enthusiastic about telephone consultations. This stemmed from their strong conviction that nothing could replace the direct doctor-patient relationship. Any limitations on direct contact might increase the risk of misdiagnosis. Despite these objections, men did acknowledge some potential benefits if it meant one could consult one's own GP by phone. Older men expressed the opinion that doctors themselves would be opposed to such a possibility, fearful of offering a misdiagnosis over the phone: '*Doctors would often like to see a patient before the diagnosis. Telephone consultations do not guarantee perfect exchange of information between a patient and a doctor. The patient is often not precise in defining his medical problem. Also symptoms may be similar for different diseases*'.

Telemedicine

The prospect of telemedicine did not arouse great interest among participants in the focus groups. Their observations mirrored those on telephone consultations – i.e. most doubted the effectiveness of indirect consultations and pointed to potential resistance on the part of doctors wary of misdiagnosis: *'It is not possible for telemedicine to provide sufficient contact. The patient would have to have professional medical equipment in order to be able to give precise information about their health condition'*. The only perceived advantage of telemedicine over telephone consultations was the possibility of being able to show where the pain is located, but *'the details may not be clear enough'*. All stressed the importance of the direct doctor-patient relationship that should only be given up if the doctor knows the patient and their medical history well. Contacting a doctor on a video telephone was not considered suitable in emergencies when a direct consultation is needed. A few participants suggested telemedicine might be used for psychotherapy.

EXTENDING THE SCOPE OF MEDICAL CARE

Complementary therapies

Old and new 'medicines' coexist in Poland. Improved awareness of health issues, contacts with doctors and the influence of the mass media have encouraged use of new drugs but older methods such as herbalism and self-care have remained, especially in the case of diseases that are difficult to cure.[20] The coexistence of complementary medicines alongside more conventional treatments was viewed with approval.

Recent surveys have confirmed that complementary medicine is still gaining in popularity. In 1997 around a third of Poles (35 per cent) used alternative medicine, while in 1998 this proportion had increased to 57 per cent. Polish people tend to believe that physicians should cooperate with bio-energy therapists to make treatment more effective. The general view is that unconventional methods will not harm anybody even though they may not help much either. Herbalism and chiropractic remedies are very popular, homeopathy less so.[21] Interest in alternative medicine extends to all social classes. Its popularity can be traced to the recent social and cultural transformations in Poland and an opening up to global trends. The mass media began to present aspects of new age thinking which promoted the benefits of a more holistic approach than conventional medicine.

Complementary treatments are seen as meeting the psychological needs of patients better. The values promoted by alternative therapies, such as vitality, purification of the body, positive thinking and acceptance of natural remedies are now well established in patients' minds.[20] However, some focus group participants were more sceptical: *'Unfortunately alternative therapists do not always have professional experience and they can worsen the condition of a particular patient'.*

Views were related to experience. Those who had tried alternative therapies usually had a positive attitude towards them, but they tended to distinguish between treatments like herbal medicine or chiropractic approaches, which were seen as reliable, and others like bioenergotherapy (mind over matter), which were not. There was a general view that complementary alternatives should always be discussed with a doctor. Participants felt that patients should always inform their doctors if they were using such treatments.

New medicines and biotechnologies

Genetic testing can provide early diagnosis and permit the implementation of effective treatment. Patients in the focus groups felt that the more serious the illness the more justified the use of these tests. It was recognized that early diagnosis may prevent the development of certain medical conditions such as cancer, diabetes, heart disease and allergies: *'Such tests could prevent the development of the disease; speed is often necessary in diagnosing and treatment'.*

Male participants were positive about the possibility of self-diagnosis tests as long as they are reliable and cheap. Women tended to be more cautious, saying these tests should only be offered by those who are medically competent. Results should be strictly confidential to prevent them from getting into the wrong hands: *'Such tests should be done by authorized professionals, they should not be publicly available, and should obviously be protected with a code'.*

While it was believed that knowledge about a predisposition to certain conditions may trigger appropriate prophylactic measures and motivate patients to fight the illness, women patients feared that such knowledge could have a major psychological impact. They therefore felt it was important to agree standards for the way in which such information is given to patients. Women felt the assistance of a psychologist might be necessary, whereas men considered patient reaction to this information to be a secondary issue:

'When we are terminally ill, we may become mentally weaker, but if we learn about the possibility of an illness in advance, we may try to prevent it'.

One negative aspect of genetic testing mentioned by participants was the possibility of a perceived 'death sentence' changing the patient's personality and natural behaviour.

Attitudes to prenatal tests are affected by the standpoint taken by the Catholic Church. In May 1999 the Polish Parliament passed certain legal amendments that severely restricted access to prenatal tests while extending the protection of the foetus. This sparked a fierce debate in the mass media, especially the press. Polls revealed that 88 per cent of Poles felt that women have a right to prenatal tests, despite the risks they may present to the foetus.[22]

The majority felt the new restrictions were wrong. Positive attitudes to prenatal tests do not necessarily imply agreement that a foetus can be aborted if there is a risk of disability, but the vast majority of respondents felt that the tests should be available even if the risks (e.g. of miscarriage) might be increased.

INFORMATION FOR PATIENTS

Health information needs

The implementation of the health care reforms created an increased demand for information on issues such as how to choose a GP, accessing a specialist and health insurance documentation. Only 7 per cent of Poles said they fully understood the implications of the reforms. More than half felt uninformed, with 39 per cent saying they 'hardly understood' these principles and 20 per cent claiming to be 'totally confused'[4] Not surprisingly, this was related to educational level. Individuals with a university education felt better informed than people with only an elementary or secondary education. Older people and those with only an elementary education complained about lack of information, stressing the need for better information about specialist and rehabilitation services, and out-patient rehabilitation centres.[5]

Above all, patients want information about how to look after themselves after discharge from hospital, including dietary advice, advice on recommended activity levels and on what to do if a disease relapses or other worrying symptoms appear. Information about health status was seen as one of the worst aspects of inpatient care.[23]

Young people, qualified labourers and individuals with vocational education were particularly dissatisfied with the information provided on health status and treatment.[24] It was not recognized as a problem by respondents with a university or elementary education.

Annual surveys indicate a gradual but slow improvement in understanding about how to access health services in the new system. The subjective feeling of being informed was a decisive factor influencing people's opinion about the reforms. Those who felt better informed had more positive opinions of the health care system and the quality of health services.[25]

Patients in the focus groups wanted information about their illness, health status, prognosis, the side-effects of treatment (including negative ones) and nutrition. Female patients in particular said they expected clear and understandable information on the health care system, but they expected health professionals to provide this: *'A doctor should be informed about any changes in health services so as to be able to provide adequate answers when questioned'.*

Participants wanted more detailed information about treatment options, hospital quality and the performance of individual health professionals. They also wanted information about the availability and costs of alternative or complementary medicine.

Women in the focus groups wanted their doctors to provide a range of information and to create the kind of atmosphere that helps patients talk freely about their health problems and about prevention: *'Doctors should pay more attention to our bad habits . . . provide health information on losing weight, advise smokers on how to give up smoking etc.'*

Men seemed less anxious to ask their doctors questions but they claimed to establish better contact with nurses. Participants felt that information should always be provided in a full and accessible form. Younger women in particular said that they were proactive in looking for information about their health, the side-effects of drugs and cheaper drug alternatives.

Information sources

The focus group research indicated that women tended to seek information from friends and relatives and from the media before they saw a doctor. Although they looked for answers to their questions, they were sceptical about what they found, especially the younger age group. Young women sought health information from their beautician who advised them on their skin problems and from their dietician who advised them on their eating habits. Women regarded this kind of problem as too minor to discuss with a doctor.

For older men, the main sources of health information were friends and relatives. The younger age group willingly used the media – newspapers, magazines, radio, television and the internet – although they also valued the opinions of their family and friends.

Gender was an important factor in determining views about the reliability of health information. Women were more likely to trust specialists, their GPs and nurses. Men had more confidence in their family and friends. There was some scepticism about the media as a source of health information. Media reports were felt to focus on negative issues and to distort the facts. Information provided by doctors was seen as much more reliable.

Health websites

Medical websites are now one of the ways of promoting health and patient-oriented education. IKAR was one of the first health promotion websites that provided information on heart disease, the major cause of death in Poland. It consists of two parts: Patient Education and Preventing Cardiovascular Diseases. Patients who are interested may find information on diagnostics (how to prepare for medical examination; possible discomfort caused by diagnostic equipment; indications to be followed), heart surgery (how to get ready for surgery; preoperative, operative and postoperative measures) and prevention.[26] Other websites are available on allergies, obesity, influenza and diabetes, and the amount of information on the internet is growing fast.

The internet has not yet become a very popular source of medical knowledge for Polish patients. Only 16 per cent of survey respondents reported having access to the internet at home or at work.[27] Poles appreciate quick access to information via the internet, but they are anxious that it may adversely affect personal and interpersonal contacts, and give children and young people easy access to pornography and violent computer games.

Some health care centres have begun to disseminate health information by creating internet cafes for patients within the framework of the European Commission project, the Patient Internet Cafe.[28] For most people this is usually their first contact with the internet, though at least 50 per cent have some previous experience with computers. Internet cafes in health care centres, especially in rehabilitation units, provide information about diseases and have a therapeutic function as they help people forget about their suffering and promote communication with others.

Several focus group participants reported using the internet to search for information concerning health centres, doctors, medicines (cheaper alternative drugs), and advice on how to act in emergencies. Those with chronic diseases wanted information about self-help groups and rehabilitation centres. Younger women with children searched for information about new treatments and drugs so as to be able to discuss them later with a doctor: '*I expect to find on the web information concerning health problems, treatment, health centres that specialize in curing certain disorders. Searching the internet is much quicker than in the library*'.

But there was a strong feeling that the internet is not a very reliable source of information. People complained that nobody really verifies the information on the websites and it is difficult to find the relevant information. It was considered particularly important to know the sources of information provided on health websites.

PATIENT EMPOWERMENT

Self-diagnosis, self-medication, self-care

For less serious illnesses, self-medication is very popular among Polish patients. Some 65 per cent of patients reported using self-medication to treat conditions such as colds, headaches, stomach pains and food poisoning.[19] According to a recent survey, 40 per cent of Poles rely on home remedies or a combination of pharmacological drugs and home remedies.[21]

Focus group participants had no problems in listing the factors that determine a healthy lifestyle. Younger respondents mentioned sport and education first, whereas the older age group emphasized nutrition and the avoidance of bad habits, especially cigarette smoking. A healthy diet was believed to consist of fruit and vegetables and a small amount of meat and cholesterol. Fruit and vegetables (including the miraculous garlic) were seen as good sources of natural vitamins; their consumption was believed to be better than supplementing one's diet with synthetic vitamins. Excessive dieting was thought to result in anaemia and anorexia: '*We can help ourselves if we don't regard ourselves wiser than the doctors. If we are on a diet and are not careful enough, it could lead to anaemia or anorexia*'.

Older patients often mentioned a lack of stress as a factor that contributes to good health. A healthy lifestyle was also understood to include regular check-ups, particularly for women. It was considered to be the patient's responsibility to take all prescribed medications and adhere to recommended rehabilitation programmes.

Participants felt it was the patient's responsibility to eat an appropriate diet, attend consultations and have regular check-ups, take regular exercise, reduce the intake of stimulants (e.g. coffee and alcohol) and give up smoking, avoid stress wherever possible and take vitamin supplements. Generally, people viewed medicine as a useful tool in the diagnostic and treatment process but felt they had responsibility for their own health.

Involvement in treatment decisions

Not discussed.

Electronic patient-held records

In discussing likely future developments in health care, the most popular scenario presented to focus group participants was the prospect of storing an individual's medical history on a smart card. Participants liked this idea, but only on the condition that personal data would be well protected from unauthorized access. Patients stressed the universal character of the card, its usefulness while travelling, in emergencies and accidents, and greater precision and accuracy in transmitting data. The possibility of transmitting comprehensive information was particularly valued: *'It's a good idea because smart cards would save time. The patient wouldn't have to tell his whole medical history'*.

Older patients felt that smart cards could give them more information about their own medical histories: *'Each patient would have the possibility to access his medical history any time he wishes to do so'*.

There was concern amongst some of the younger group members that smart cards would need particularly strong data protection mechanisms. They were especially concerned about possible access by insurance companies, arguing that only doctors and emergency services should have access to the card.

Choosing where to receive care

Teaching hospitals and tertiary referral centres are located in cities where there are medical schools. There are 11 such centres for nearly

40 million people. Therefore, on average, one centre serves about 9 million people. This means that many patients have to commute, sometimes travelling 100km for treatment. There are several specialist hospital centres used by patients from all over Poland, such as the Child Care Centre or the Institute of Haematology in Warsaw.

The idea of providing comprehensive, national information disseminated through the mass media about doctors and health centres was welcomed by focus group participants who thought it would be very helpful when choosing a doctor or specialist. It was felt that the publication of information about the quality of health services would impose a form of continuous quality control on doctors and health institutions: *'Better health centres set higher standards, thus forcing the worse ones to improve quality of health services and adapt to the best practice'.*

Patients were aware of the difficulties and limitations of attempting to create a league table of the best doctors and health sites. Such a scheme could have drawbacks – the best doctors and health centres would be in too much demand as *'everyone cannot be treated by a few health professionals in a few health centres'.* Some group members doubted the reliability of such rankings. They believed that the professional associations would exert considerable influence and incompetence would seldom be acknowledged. In order to be objective and reliable, it was felt that information about quality should be collected by an independent body unconnected with health professionals or medical associations.

NEW ROLES FOR THE CITIZEN

Strengthening patients' rights

The gradual move from a paternalistic to a partnership model in Poland has been manifested in health legislation and in patients' attitudes and expectations. In the 1990s several acts were passed to guarantee patients' rights, including the Constitution of the Republic of Poland, the Healthcare Organizations Act of 1996, the Medical Profession Act of 1996, the Mental Healthcare Act, and a number of other acts and decrees. Legal and ethical regulations applicable under Polish law define such matters as the patient's right to agree or disagree to medical treatment, the right to be informed about their health status, to have access to medical records, as well as the right to patient privacy, protection of personal data, respect for dignity and freedom of will. Patients are also protected by regulations included in the Medical Ethics Code.[29] All regulations relating to the patient's status in the health care system are brought together in the so-called Charter of Patient's Rights.[30]

Officially, therefore, the rights of patients seem well protected. Five years ago, Polish patients' awareness of their rights and duties was poor. In a survey carried out in 1996, two fifths of respondents had never heard of such rights, nearly half had heard about them but had very limited knowledge and few were aware that patients are protected by law.[26] Several instances were reported where patients' rights had been ignored. For example, 51 per cent of survey respondents complained they had had to pay for medicines which should have been free for inpatients, 43 per cent reported that they had been pressurized to seek private treatment, 30 per cent said their inpatient care lacked privacy, and others complained of limited time for visitors in hospitals, lack of information about treatment, lack of opportunity to give consent for treatment methods and failure to inform them about their right to access to their medical records.[24]

However, participants in our focus groups had no difficulty in recognizing their rights. Younger people stressed the importance of freedom to choose doctors and health centres, and older patients considered access to a doctor, particularly a specialist, an absolute right. The rights to information about their own health, drugs, alternative forms of treatment and a second opinion were considered to be among the most important: *'A doctor should recommend another specialist or another treatment so that a patient could have a right to choose'.*

Opinions on patient safety and malpractice were rather varied. Almost one in three survey respondents could identify examples of malpractice or negligence. Typically, patients mention such errors as wrong diagnosis (17 per cent), errors in the treatment of children (11 per cent) and inappropriate hospital treatment (medical errors, bad diagnosis based on test results).[12] But generally, Poles are of the opinion that malpractice happens rarely – two thirds of respondents said that health professionals make errors occasionally or rarely. Most Poles trust health professionals and physicians are accorded high social status. Surveyed about their probable reaction to a case of malpractice, the most frequent response would be to lodge a complaint with a medical court (64 per cent), claim damages in legal proceedings (60 per cent) or lodge a complaint with the sick fund (58 per cent). Some 64 per cent of respondents believed that the chances of getting compensation would be almost nil, while most of those who had experience of claiming damages admitted that it was very difficult.[31]

Participation in policy making

Nowadays Poles are more conscious of the payments they make to the various sick funds than they were of paying taxes under the old system of financing health care. This makes them feel they have a greater right to demand appropriate medical services.[5] An organized movement of health care consumers, as seen in some other European countries, has not yet emerged in Poland but patients' involvement in policy decisions, though still not widespread, seems to be on the increase. Self-help groups have begun to organize with the support of governmental organizations. Groups exist for patients with rheumatic disease, multiple sclerosis and breast cancer, and for mental health service users. Representatives of these groups take part in conferences and workshops and even participate in legislative activities.

In August 1994, representatives of non-governmental organizations and experts were asked to participate in the work of the Parliamentary Commission on the Mental Health Act. They were expected to provide input relating to the organization of self-help centres and the running of self-help groups in mental health. The importance and significance of self-help groups is expected to grow.[32] However, it takes time to translate declarations on patient involvement into reality. Cooperation between self-help groups and the sick funds has so far been reflected in the statute of only one of the sick funds.

Table 5.1 The focus groups in the Polish study

Group	No. of partici- pants	Age	Sex	Location	Health status
1	8	18–40	Male	Kraków	Out- or inpatient, healthy
2	10	18–40	Female	Kraków	Out- or inpatient, healthy
3	8	41–65	Male	Kraków	Inpatient, chronic illness
4	10	41–65	Female	Kraków	Inpatient, chronic illness

FOCUS GROUPS

Focus groups were run between 8th and 9th August and on 4th of September 2001. Details of each group are shown in Table 5.1.

NOTES

1 Public Opinion Research Centre (CBOS) (2000) *Opinions on the Healthcare System After Two Years of Reforms.* Warsaw: CBOS.
2 Main Statistical Office (1999) *Healthcare in Households.* Warsaw: Main Statistical Office.
3 Ryiko, E. (1998) *Opinions on Outpatient Units and Hospitals – A Report from Qualitative Research.* Kraków: Marketing Research Centre.
4 Jędrzejewski, M. and Kamiński, P. (1999) *Patients' Opinions on Medical Services.* Unpublished report.
5 Halik, J., Borkowska-Kalwas, T. and Pączkowska, M. (1999) *Assessment of Availability of Medical Services.* Unpublished report.
6 Tokarski, S. (1999) Health service reform in the opinions of inhabitants and health service personnel in the Lublin Province, *Zdrowie Publiczne*, 10.
7 Rozum, Z. (1997) Patients' expectations from family doctors and GPs and possibilities of their realisation on the basis of a survey conducted in Żywiec, *Problemy Medycyny*, 32.
8 Public Opinion Research Centre (CBOS) (2000) *Healthcare – A Responsibility of the State or the Citizens?* Warsaw: CBOS.
9 Public Opinion Research Centre (CBOS) (2000) *Reducing Payments for Medical Treatment.* Warsaw: CBOS.
10 Public Opinion Research Centre (CBOS) (2000) *Egalitarians in Polish Society.* Warsaw: CBOS.
11 *Statistical Yearbook* (2000) Warsaw: Zaklad Wydawnictw Statystycznych (ZWS).
12 Public Opinion Research Centre (CBOS) (2001) *Medical Errors and Confidence in Doctors.* Warsaw: CBOS.
13 Gaertner, H. (1997) Doctor, patient and empathy, in *Medicine at the Beginning of the 21st Century: Doctor's Personality as a Remedy.* Warsaw: Polska Akademia Medyeyny.
14 Lęczyca Healthcare Organization (2000) *Patients' Satisfaction Survey.* Kraków: Łęczyca Healthcare Organization.
15 Marć, M. (2000) Interpersonal communication and the level of patients' and families' satisfaction with nursing care, in *Fifth Conference 'Quality in Healthcare'.* Kraków: NCQA.
16 Kulczycka, K. (1999) Patients' opinions on quality of nursing care, in *Fourth Conference: 'Quality in Healthcare'.* Kraków: NCQA.
17 Glowacka, M. and Bukowska, A. (1998) Patients' satisfaction with nursing care in hospitals, *Zdrowie i Zarządzanie*, Report 2.

18 Walewski, P. (2001) Kwadratowe pigulki (The Square Pills), *Polityka*, 9 June.
19 Bartkowiak, L. (1997). Pharmacy in the eyes of patients, *Problemy Medycyny Spolecznej*, 32: 615–16.
20 Piątkowski, W. (1999) Non-medical treatment as a method of cultural interpretation, *Annales Universitatis Mariae Curie-Sklodowska*, 7: 111–17.
21 Piatkowski, W. (1998) The necessity for sociological studies on non-professional ways of catering for health needs in a pluralistic society, in A. Sulek (ed.) *Silesia – Poland – Europe: Changing Society in a Local and Global Perspective*. Katowice: Wydawnictwo University.
22 Public Opinion Research Centre (CBOS) (1999) *Current Problems and Events: Opinions on Prenatal Tests*. Warsaw: CBOS.
23 National Centre for Quality Assessment in Healthcare (NCQA) (2000) *Reports from Surveys Conducted in Hospitals*. Kraków: NCQA.
24 Public Opinion Research Centre (CBOS) (1996) *'Omnibus' Research Project*. CBOS.
25 Public Opinion Research Centre (CBOS) (2000) *Opinions on the Functioning of the Healthcare System*. Warsaw: CBOS.
26 ICAR (ICARUS): a web program promoting health for patients, http://nadcisnienie.pl/konference/prace/ikar.html.
27 Internet information about Demoskop survey, 2000, taken from website www.onet.pl.
28 The Patient Internet Cafe (PIC) Project was implemented in 1999 in the Silesian Rehabilitation Centre in Ustronie.
29 Krzak, M. (1999) Protection of patient's rights in the light of inter-national law and Polish legislation, *Antidotum*, 6–7: 29–82.
30 Bielewicz, A. (1998) The charter of patient rights, *Służba zdrowia*, Report no. 103–105.
31 Public Opinion Research Centre (CBOS) (2000) *Opinions on the Potential Requirements of Poles*. Warsaw: CBOS.
32 Bobiatyńska, E. (1999) Co-ordination models in healthcare and welfare systems, *Zdrowie Publiczne* (supplement).

6

SLOVENIA

OPINIONS ABOUT THE HEALTH CARE SYSTEM

The present system

Slovenia underwent considerable socioeconomic and political change in the period 1988–1991. Parliamentary democracy was established with the first multiparty elections in 1990 and independence was declared on 25 June 1991. Health care reform was one of the first important developments. It began before independence and was completed shortly after. New health care legislation was adopted in 1992. The most important changes included the introduction of a health insurance system with universal coverage regulated by the Health Insurance Institute of Slovenia (HIIS), the introduction of private provision of health care and the establishment of health professionals' chambers.

The national health care programme was adopted in June 2000, after seven years of debate. Concessions are granted by the local communities for primary health care and by the Ministry of Health for all other types of services in health care. Legal delays in granting new concessions meant that more deprived areas could only acquire additional services at the expense of patients themselves. Out of hours non-emergency care is provided by primary health care centres, which organize care for their catchment area. This is provided either through the organized efforts of the health centre physicians alone or in collaboration with the private providers of care.

Pre-hospital units are a key component of the project, which is reorganizing emergency medical services in the entire territory of Slovenia.[1] At specially regulated locations, trained teams capable of providing emergency care are now available. A physician and other health professionals are on standby. The plan is for calls to the general emergency number to be triaged by a professional who would be able to counsel callers and provide professional support to the pre-hospital team in cases of accidents and injury. The units work closely with the fire brigade and other rescue teams on the ground. Like primary health centres, these units are on the lowest organizational rung of the health service structure. Funding is a particular problem as all costs are charged in full to the HIIS.

Access and responsiveness

Slovenia has a longstanding tradition of population surveys, dating back to the beginning of the 1980s. In the years 1994, 1996 and 1999 three special surveys were run parallel to the general survey, 'Slovene Public Opinion', with specific questions about health and health care, including questions on general levels of satisfaction.[2] In 1999, one third of respondents were not satisfied with the services provided and only a quarter were very satisfied. More worryingly, over 40 per cent said they did not believe that the health service would provide them with the best possible treatment when needed. Private health care was seen as offering better quality, although the proportion of those who feel it is better has decreased over time. People are most satisfied with the services provided by GPs and dentists and much less so with those provided by medical specialists. About one third of those surveyed had seen their GP once or twice over the previous year and 10 per cent had seen their GP ten or more times over the previous year.

The Slovene Public Opinion Survey reported waiting times for medical specialists, dentists and GPs. The problem of long waits was worst for medical specialists (33 per cent had to wait six months or more).[2] It is encouraging, however, that about 36 per cent of specialists' patients and about a half of dental patients did not have to wait at all. Asked how long they had waited to be seen by their GP, one third of those surveyed in a primary health centre answered that it was between 15 and 30 minutes, while 22 per cent waited more than an hour. Waiting times at walk-in clinics were longer with 14 per cent of GP patients reporting waits of more than two hours, but as many as 20 per cent had to wait that long at a specialist's office. Reasons for long waits include staff maternity and sickness leave, and postgraduate training absences.

In-clinic waiting times in primary care vary, but making appointments for a specific time has become the norm recently. Another frequently used option is the split day, in which one part is dedicated to patients with acute illnesses, while patients with chronic conditions and older patients are called for appointments later in the day. Specialist outpatient visits are a much bigger problem. Waiting times vary among specialties and between regions. Problems arose when personal physicians started to refer increasing numbers of patients to specialists. It has also become common practice for specialists to arrange follow-up appointments. An effort has been made to standardize appointment procedures in the hope that waiting times can be reduced to a maximum of one week.

Triage systems, together with afternoon shifts, have helped to reduce unnecessary follow-up visits and have led to a reduction in waiting times. Extremely long waiting times in thyroid disease specialties were a consequence of an unregulated system of reimbursement for hormone tests. Since these tests were reimbursable only to specialists, not GPs, the latter simply referred their patients to specialists who were obliged to see all patients with a referral form. Since the HIIS started reimbursing GPs for these services, only patients in real need of specialist examinations are referred and waiting times have been reduced by several months.

There has been a significant reduction in waiting times for cardiology, urology and endocrinology, but less reduction in time spent waiting to see orthopaedic surgeons and ENT. The parallel management of patients by GPs and specialists is being tried in orthopaedics and bowel disease. If the pilot schemes produce good results, then the system will be extended to other areas. People with psychiatric problems have free access to their personal physician and also to their psychiatrist. Since there is no requirement for a GP to refer patients for psychiatric treatment, there are no constraints on the free use of the entire service.

The focus groups were concerned that access is hampered by the various mechanisms to reduce demand. Patients perceived these as a serious obstacle to the health care they need. Some participants pointed to important regional differences which drive patients to seek care in the larger cities: '*Well, I don't like the fact that in a provincial health care centre one cannot get referred to the lab as often as that happens in Ljubljana'*.

People feel strongly that access is one of the basic principles of equity in health care. This was illustrated throughout the debate in the 1990s by resistance to hospital closures on the one hand and demands for even more primary health care centres on the other. Following all these debates, no hospital was closed down (although some reduced their bed numbers) and two new primary health care centres were established.

Structure and organization

Several changes have been introduced in the way in which hospitals are financed. The aim is to achieve a better distribution of limited funds, collected through compulsory insurance contributions, among the hospitals in Slovenia. Some of the less well-resourced hospitals are guaranteed a certain level of funding by the HIIS under the new reimbursement scheme, but others have to negotiate.

In 1998 the first phase of the so-called standardization of hospital care began. This set lengths of stay in hospitals according to the number of people using each hospital. It is an agreed method by which the anticipated funds for salaries, running costs, decommissioning and other expenses are distributed among regional hospitals. The most important new initiative is the Health Sector Management Project to be financed partly through a loan from the World Bank.[3] The project should help to reform hospital management and reimbursement systems through a better decision making process.

In Slovenia there are approximately 1800 inhabitants per primary care physician.[4] There are regions, however, where the ratio is much less healthy, rising to more than 2000 or even 3000 inhabitants per physician. These regions include several in the north and north-east like Koroska, Prekmurje and Kozjansko, the regions of Ptuj and Ormoz, and Tolmin in the west. The European average is about 1600 inhabitants per physician. An average physician's office in Slovenia has 40 visits per day, while the average in the EU has about 20.

There is a shortage of physicians and dentists in primary care. A large number of physicians are near retirement age while many younger doctors are choosing to work in the pharmaceutical industry or elsewhere outside of the medical profession. Many physicians are on specialist training which means they are absent from surgeries for most of the four-year training period. The remainder are unevenly distributed and too concentrated in the big cities and in the capital, Ljubljana.

The shortage of doctors is most obvious in the remote rural areas of the north-east and north-west. The median age of doctors in these areas is over 50, which means that about half will retire in the next ten years.[5] For the whole of Slovenia this means that 500 new primary care physicians are needed over the next ten years, or 50 a year. The annual intake to general practice is only about 10 to 15 per year. In the future, additional shortages are expected if specialization in family medicine is to become an addition to the extended internship period rather than part of the regular training. The main danger of the new system lies in the fact that physicians in training will now have to spend much more time working in hospitals instead of slowly moving into primary care. This will lead to longer absences from GP work where help was expected at least on a combined basis. These problems threaten the future functioning of rural surgeries, prevention and on-call services.

There was an impression among focus group participants that primary care services are not organized efficiently and that health professionals do not respect patients' time: *'We are under more and more pressure at our workplace to be punctual and precise at what we do. People in health care should understand that they have to respect that and that we are not able to come only in the mornings, but they should adapt their schedules, too'.*

Several participants claimed that the appointment system works against the acutely ill and favours people with chronic conditions who usually cope better with waiting. They also thought that unfairness was introduced through the use of personal contacts. Some believed that the increasing unfairness and inequity of the health care system was an extension of similar trends in many other countries. Many people felt that patients have to invest too much time, energy and money whenever they enter the health care system. health care providers should give greater consideration to patient needs for flexibility of access in non-emergency cases: *'I don't like having to make an appointment. I wish I could come whenever I feel the need for a check-up'.*

Recent developments that were viewed more positively included the introduction of the personal physician concept (i.e. GP), which enables easier and less formal doctor-patient interaction, smart cards and shorter waiting times in GP surgeries.

Cost and efficiency

Health insurance introduced universal coverage. People who have no personal incomes are registered with local communities who provide for the payment of the compulsory insurance benefit package. This is loosely defined, which can cause difficulties. The benefits available under the scheme are described in the *Rules and Standing Orders of Compulsory Health Insurance*, issued by the HIIS.

The establishment of the HIIS and separation of funding from the national budget were seen as important steps towards financial stability. In 1992 insurance contributions increased steeply, with the proportion of gross salaries dedicated to health care rising to an astonishing 18 per cent. The rate was reduced in 1996 to 13.5 per cent, which still ensures stable financing. But voluntary or supplementary health insurance now accounts for almost 15 per cent of all health care funds. These supplementary payments are based on flat-rate premiums rather than income-related contributions. There is some evidence of cream-skimming since the first private insurance company to offer this type of insurance recruited predominantly younger people.

Public attitudes towards changes in health care financing are somewhat ambivalent, especially in respect of higher private contributions. Of respondents to the Slovene Public Opinion Survey,[2] 40 per cent were not convinced by the statement that an individual would take better care of their health if they pay more out of their own pocket or voluntary insurance. Almost half of those surveyed said it is unfair for the state to put a bigger financial burden on patients. Income-related rights in health care are a similarly controversial issue. There is still a strong sense of solidarity within the population: 77 per cent of those surveyed said that premiums should not be age-related. About 40 per cent felt that people who indulge in dangerous sporting activities (parachuting, mountaineering etc.) should pay higher premiums, while 46 per cent thought they should not.

In 1999 only 3 per cent of survey respondents reported problems with their compulsory health insurance. This represents a significant reduction since 1994 when problems were reported by 12 per cent. Slightly more than half (53 per cent) of the insured said they would complain if they were dissatisfied with their health insurance, but about half of those felt the HIIS complaint procedures were not well organized. A similar proportion was critical of the voluntary insurers' complaint procedures. Efforts have been underway to define new reimbursement methods. A proposed increase in the contribution rate was opposed both by contributors and by the Ministry of Finance. Instead, they felt that the collection of contributions could be organized more efficiently.

The financial health of all the major health care providers has been the centre of attention for years now. Three hospitals have received particular attention. The main hospital of the country, the Clinical Centre of Ljubljana, continues to suffer major financial losses and regional hospitals in Izola and Celje have also faced serious problems.

Salaries of health professionals remain the focus of debate. Physicians and dentists won significant salary increases following a strike in 1996 and physicians are now among the best-paid professionals in the country. Nurses received a significantly smaller increase and it is difficult to recruit non-medical personnel. There are already several hospitals in Slovenia that have no pharmacists.

In focus group discussions patients complained that the HIIS is excluding more and more medications from the list of approved drugs. The cost of these drugs is not refundable. This is a big burden for the elderly who suffer from chronic diseases, have relatively low incomes and cannot always afford co-payments.

Equity

Patients are increasingly assuming responsibility for their own health through healthier lifestyles, but they also have to bear a bigger financial burden in terms of treatment costs. Long waiting times in certain services, particularly gynaecology, dentistry and ophthalmology (mainly due to a lack of physicians) have led to the establishment of special surgeries to provide services for direct payment within guidelines set by the Ministry of Health. For those who can pay, this allows direct access to a specialist with little or no waiting time. Some 25 per cent of patients use private providers for medical or dental care, and 40 per cent of these choose to pay for the services directly even though they could probably get them for free as part of the compulsory insurance package. The main point of concern is the lack of equity in such a system. Half of all survey respondents objected to the reintroduction of co-payments.[2]

Another problem of the Slovene health system is that resource distribution and physician payment systems tend to favour younger and healthier people, with less going to older people and those who are seriously ill. For example, the HIIS ensures that doctors are paid regardless of the number of patient visits. The most expensive patients are those aged 60 and above but current incentives do not adequately reflect the changing demographic situation.

Kersnik carried out a study to establish whether patients from various ethnic backgrounds are treated differently by their personal physicians.[6] He found that overall satisfaction was slightly lower in non-native speaking patients (83.6 vs. 85.8 points). Ethnic minority patients were less satisfied with physicians' thoroughness, their ability to relieve symptoms quickly and to explain the nature of particular illnesses. In multivariate analysis, Slovene nationality predicted higher patient satisfaction with physicians' clinical behaviour.

The qualitative research suggested that access to health care is getting worse each year. A frequent observation from the focus groups was that too many services – even those that patients feel entitled to under compulsory insurance – now have to be paid for, in full or in part. There was also an awareness of the rather ruthless influence of private practice. Participants felt that they got better access to many services when paying out-of-pocket: '*If you need physiotherapy you have to go to a private provider. If you want these services to be paid from health insurance, you have to wait for treatment for at least six months*'.

The focus group participants were generally not very optimistic about future trends. They saw the increase in out-of-pocket expenses continuing. Younger men seemed to be very pragmatic about this, but younger and middle-aged women worried about how they would cope. Older men were especially critical, reflecting on all the years they contributed to health care funds. All groups shared the opinion that in future, access to many services would depend on the patient's ability to pay. While all age groups saw this as inevitable, they still believed the state should intervene to limit potential inequity. Several patients said that if they had to pay for drugs they would only buy them in an emergency.

PATIENTS' VIEWS OF HEALTH PROFESSIONALS

Doctors

Trust in doctors is very high in Slovenia. According to the Slovene Public Opinion Survey, only about 9 per cent of those who use GP services are uncertain about whether the treatment provided for them is optimal.[2] However, 5 per cent of patients reported that certain types of treatment are available only on payment of a fee directly to the doctor, suggesting a certain level of corruption.

In one of a series of studies of patients' views on the quality of GP services, Kersnik surveyed 2160 patients attending 36 family practices in Slovenia.[7] Almost three out of five patients felt the care they received was excellent. The highest level of reported problems concerned waiting times in the surgery. The three characteristics on which patients made the most favourable observations were: confidentiality of records, the ability of GPs to listen to their patients and their accessibility by phone. A recent study compared the levels of satisfaction expressed by Slovene patients with those in other European countries.[8] Slovene doctors showed less interest in patients' personal problems and were less likely to talk informally with them. They scored particularly well on accessibility, confidentiality and response to emergency situations. They scored less well on issues which also caused dissatisfaction elsewhere – i.e. the management of emotional problems, information about the possible outcome of specialist referrals and waiting times.

A further study looked at patients' main reasons for choosing a GP.[9] It found that 70 per cent of patients chose a physician they knew beforehand. For 14 per cent of patients, the recommendation of relatives and friends was crucial. Three qualities were identified as the most important: that their physician takes time for their problems (91 per cent), that they have expert knowledge (88 per cent) and that they are friendly and kind (75 per cent). The willingness to carry out home visits was also important in making the choice.

Kersnik's survey found that patients tended to choose to stay with a particular surgery because they had had a positive experience there and 60 per cent were very satisfied with the treatment they received from their GP.[7] It seems that patients are in general satisfied with the services provided by GPs. Most have become quite faithful to their doctors and are unhappy if they are absent for a long period of time.

In general, focus group participants had an ambivalent attitude towards their physicians. On the one hand they agreed that doctors deserved the substantial salary increases they had received over the last five years – '*It is very important what your GP is like. He is the first person you contact when you get ill. He knows everything about you, and does the best for you. He is the person you trust*' – but on the other hand they had higher expectations of doctors and the system. Many focus group participants did not feel that their GPs communicated with them satisfactorily, leaving them to ask questions rather than offering explanations.

Participants preferred to see the same GP who knew about their problems, their medical history and their family background. They saw this as an important element in building trust and better co-operation between doctor and patient. Most of the patients would not wish to see a different doctor even if that meant that they could be seen quicker. A combination of an appointment system for chronic patients and same-day examinations for the acutely ill or those with a newly-presented problem seemed the most popular solution:

> *If you need a doctor and there is someone else you don't know and he doesn't know you, you cannot be confident with him. Of course, there is a possibility that he is a good doctor, but you never know.*

> *If you have toothache, you don't mind if there is another dentist that relieves your pain.'*

Nurses

Nursing quality assurance projects are running in some hospitals. The main goal is the introduction of a system which produces quality nursing, a comprehensive approach to patient management, a higher level of patient satisfaction, more job satisfaction for nurses and better cost efficiency. Quality assurance is a new field, not only in nursing but also in health care as a whole. Slovenia still has a long way to go to achieve a better standard of nursing care, but overall patient satisfaction with the health care system frequently depends on the performance of nurses.

The focus group participants thought that nurses are already too overwhelmed by the administrative work they do in GP surgeries and should not be expected to do more. Some patients expressed concern about nurses' knowledge and overall competence in diagnosis. Most participants wanted to see more training for nurses and pharmacists if they are to be more actively involved in the diagnostic and therapeutic procedures of health care.

Pharmacists

An important study looked at people's perceptions of pharmacists.[10] It showed that patients are increasingly likely to seek advice, counselling and medication directly from the pharmacist. The community pharmacy has always had a crucial role in the public health system, and community pharmacists play an important part in health education and counselling.

Pharmacists were seen as easily accessible and the first line of assistance with less serious problems such as minor injuries or flu. But focus group participants were concerned about the trend for pharmacies to become shops for all sorts of goods rather than real health care institutions. Pharmacists were seen as professionals who had the most up-to-date knowledge about new drugs, frequently better than that of doctors. If there were a special consultation room and someone available (who need not necessarily be a doctor), they would trust a pharmacist to prescribe drugs for allergies, sore throats, or flu. On the other hand, it was felt that pharmacists knew little about the symptoms of more serious diseases and they might fail to diagnose these correctly. Some focus group participants had bought appropriate drugs directly from pharmacists, but in most cases pharmacists advise people to visit their doctor.

ALTERNATIVE WAYS OF ACCESSING HEALTH ADVICE

Telephone

In theory, telephone advice is available from a GP but in practice this varies a lot. Physicians often complain that this type of advice, although cost-effective and beneficial to the patient in certain circumstances, is not reflected in the financial reimbursement received. Since there is common agreement among stakeholders that this ought to be part of the service provided by GPs, it is expected that it will be reimbursed soon.

Participants in the focus groups felt reassured when they could access their doctor by telephone, although there were differences according to gender and patient category. Younger women, especially mothers, felt the need to have this option readily available at any time of the day or night so they could contact their child's paediatrician by mobile phone whenever they needed to. Some focus group participants explained how efficient such solutions were. Others, particularly men, feared that telephone consultations could interfere with the work of the physician in their surgery. They did not want their visit to be interrupted by one or several phone calls from other patients. But people felt that using a telephone to order a repeat prescription, check up on lab test results and arrange administrative details, like sickness notes, did speed up the process of care: '*It is excellent and quick. It even costs you less, both in terms of money and time. Your GP knows you so it is easy to present a problem and get a quick opinion about it*'.

Some patients were concerned that they would not be able to explain their problems as well on the telephone and that doctors might misinterpret their symptoms. There was also an obvious gap between older and younger age groups with the former wanting a more personalized approach. In such cases, the telephone was seen as a poor substitute.

Telemedicine

Telemedicine is not currently a big issue in Slovenia but it is anticipated that intense technological development and greater use of computers by patients and physicians will lead to an expansion of this in the future

Focus group participants saw telemedicine as an inevitable development, although it has not been widely accepted at the moment. They did not believe that the contact and the interaction between a physician and a patient could be replaced by a mere image on the screen. The only area where telemedicine did win some support was in cases where a second opinion was required from a distant, or even foreign, specialist. The majority were of the opinion that it would be more suitable for communication between a GP and a specialist. Furthermore, they did not see that it would significantly shorten waiting times: *'Also in communication by videolink, the doctor needs time to explain the disease to you. In that case it is better to have a physical examination. A doctor needs time for examination no matter if communication is by videolink, computer or personal examination'*.

EXTENDING THE SCOPE OF MEDICAL CARE

Complementary therapies

According to the 1999 Public Opinion Survey, one in three Slovenes have considered using alternative treatments to improve their health.[2] The most frequently used were herbs and herbal preparations (25 per cent) followed by diets and macrobiotics (24 per cent). Massage, chiropractic treatments and reflexology came third with 16 per cent. All other alternative or complementary therapies scored below 10 per cent. The use of health spas and baths is very widespread. They can be accessed through specially designed rehabilitation programmes when patients are referred to a spa resort with full reimbursement of medical and other health costs. Many people also spend their holidays in spas, especially in the summer.

The law in Slovenia does not regulate any non-medical procedures.

The official position of physicians' organizations is that such treatments should not be regarded as a provision of health care. The legal situation makes many patients reluctant to talk openly about such treatment. However, focus group participants provided some impressions of the types and spread of treatments used. GPs very rarely refer patients to alternative therapists but participants thought that in certain cases it would be useful to get advice and suggestions about alternative treatments from their physician. Patients believed that many psychosomatic and rheumatic conditions could be successfully treated by alternative methods: '*I see those people who deal with herbs and their natural derivatives as good complementary healers to the official health care. I don't trust those, though, who wave their hands over your head and pretend there is some energy flow or stuff'*.

New medicines and biotechnologies

For many years, all newborns have been screened at birth for phenylketonuria and for thyroid deficiency. A national programme of screening for cervical cancer for all women aged 30 to 60 at three-year intervals is in the process of being introduced. Until now this screening had only been offered on an ad hoc basis and mortality rates for cervical cancer have been on the increase.[4]

To date there has been no debate about genetic screening, not even among health care professionals and physicians. It is not surprising therefore that knowledge among focus group participants was still rather limited. When prompted to think about the potential options, people would opt for these tests when and if a clearly defined and successful treatment was available. If not, then most people in the focus groups were against genetic testing. Only younger women thought it would still be advantageous to know about a person's predisposition to certain illnesses.

INFORMATION FOR PATIENTS

Health information needs

None of the primary health centres in Slovenia provides an information service. Often the only information available is on orthopaedic aids and health promotion, together with leaflets from the HIIS. There is also a lack of information on patient rights.

Slovene patients rarely seek information about health problems before these become an issue in their daily life. Some focus group participants felt there was a risk of being too inquisitive about diseases: *'The more you seek a disease, the more you are likely to find one'*.

In general, the most trusted source of information was the GP. But before seeing them, most people would consult their family and/ or friends and if the final judgement were that the person should see a doctor, they would probably follow that advice. This attitude can lead to the late presentation of chronic diseases.

Information sources

In seeking accurate information about the introduction of new developments in health care, physicians are the most trusted source, since 45 per cent of those surveyed expressed full confidence in their physician's opinion.[2] In contrast 17 per cent trusted the Agency for Consumer Protection and only 3 per cent trusted the government.

Journals, magazines and the internet sometimes supplemented information from the GP. Of course, not all age groups and not all types of patient shared the same interest in health information. Older people, younger women (especially those with small children) and the chronically ill tended to be more active in seeking health information. Younger men and the fathers of small children were less concerned. The majority of these men tended to look for information only once they had fallen ill. People also stressed the importance of information exchange between doctors themselves. It was felt that this would also assist in better informing patients.

Health websites

A subjective overall impression is that, despite the prevalent use of traditional information sources, more and more people in Slovenia are using the internet for information on health-related issues. There is little objective evidence on the actual use of health websites but internet-use questionnaires show that about a quarter of all surveyed use the internet to access health-related information.

The development of the National Health Information Clearing House under the Health Sector Management Project will offer distant access to medical and other health data, initially to health professionals, but eventually to patients themselves.[3] It is anticipated that patients will be able to get information on local waiting lists, specialists' availability and the quality of various health care providers.

A search for internet health sources showed that most Slovene websites are dedicated to the promotion of alternative treatments and general health advice. There are, however, some pages that are interactive and provide the user with the possibility of asking questions that are answered by various medical specialists. A number of Slovene health care providers have websites, including the Clinical Centre of Ljubljana, several regional hospitals and many primary health centres. Commercial websites also provide general information on selected health topics and diseases such as cancer and asthma. Younger men in particular thought the internet was an easily accessible source of health-related information.

PATIENT EMPOWERMENT

Self-diagnosis, self-medication, self-care

Research into self-care was undertaken in the north-west region of Gorenjska.[11] A telephone survey of 200 randomly selected individuals found that people knew very little about self-care. About 46 per cent were convinced that it meant 'a healthy lifestyle'. Based on this finding the pharmacies in the region decided to produce a leaflet offering more information. The most commonly self-treated conditions in the region were flu and the common cold, followed by sore throats, mild to moderate pain and coughs. The study also found that people chose inappropriate treatments for several conditions due to inadequate advice from the local pharmacist, although only 2 per cent of all self-treated patients said they relied on this advice, whereas 36 per cent said they used their own judgement or relied on the advice of family and friends.

There are several active patient groups in Slovenia, particularly in the areas of diabetes, asthma, heart disease and cancer. All these have their own journals or magazines, most of which are available on the internet. They regularly discuss medical questions like the introduction of new treatments and service issues such as provision of medical aids and so on. The main line of communication usually involves an individual patient group and representatives of the HIIS.

Involvement in treatment decisions

According to the focus groups, doctors are still the preferred group of health professionals to be contacted, consulted and trusted with health-related issues. Most participants still expected a traditional paternalistic approach to doctor-patient relations. Even if certain services were to be transferred from doctors to other health professionals it was felt that doctors should make the decisions, maintaining their key role in diagnosis and treatment. They should be ready, though, to provide more extensive information about the process of care, the origin of disease and the prognosis.

Nevertheless, a survey carried out in 1998 found that many people expected to be actively involved in their treatment rather than simply following the instructions of their physician.[12] Respondents believed it was the duty of a GP to inform patients about to undergo a diagnostic procedure where they would be referred and why. Patients also wanted to be informed about this procedure and asked whether they consented to it. Once the diagnosis had been established, all treatment possibilities should be discussed.

People are generally unaware of their right to a second medical opinion in Slovenia.[12] In the Clinical Centre of Ljubljana there is a continuing project called 'Second Opinion Slovenia' that enables patients to acquire a second medical opinion. The service is free if the patient is referred within Slovenia, but for a second opinion from the USA patients have to pay themselves. Some commercial companies offer this service at a much lower price.

Electronic patient-held records

In 1997, HIIS started to replace the old insurance document with a smart card that would initially hold administrative data but would have the potential to include certain medical information as well. Health insurance cards were distributed to all insurees and to those professionals who are entitled to view and/or change data on the cards. The project was first implemented in a test region and an evaluation study on behalf of all the parties involved was carried out.[13] Before implementation, 62 per cent of the region supported smart cards; after their introduction, it reached 75 per cent. By the autumn of 2000 83 per cent of the Slovene population were favourably disposed to the use of smart cards.

Slovenia was one of the first countries in Europe to introduce health care smart cards for all its citizens. It is anticipated that these cards will provide a safe and uniform entry to the national health information system. Focus group participants welcomed the introduction of the cards and felt they should include information on allergies, vaccinations and recently prescribed drugs, or even the whole medical record. They saw this as a step towards a more rational and complete electronic management system in which patients would not need to worry about providing the doctor with comprehensive information. A few items of data, such as blood group and allergies, were seen as so important that they should be printed visibly on the card: *'They should be widely used and would have to include all data from birth on. And especially about allergies'*.

In the focus groups it was interesting to observe that only a few people were concerned about the inclusion of certain categories of sensitive data on the cards. However, participants did express concern about *access* to sensitive data on the smart card. There were conflicting views on whether to include disease risk factors. Participants felt that the HIIS should not have access to such information or administer it. They also felt it was unclear how changing risk factors could be kept up to date. In general, it was felt that the inclusion of risk factors on the card would mainly benefit the insurance companies and that they should find other ways of evaluating their customers' risks. Data on organ donation was also considered to be quite sensitive and patients were not convinced that this information would not be abused: *' Maybe it would be necessary to have two cards – one with some general data, of importance to various doctors and even some other health professionals; and the other with more delicate data, like a total patient history or something'; 'The point is who would use all that information – insurance companies or doctors?'*

Choosing where to receive care

Many Slovene patients choose not to use their local hospitals. Certain hospitals have to accept more patients than anticipated in the contract with the HIIS and they regulate patient numbers by reducing the length of stay. The rural areas lose most patients, since people with health insurance are entitled to a free choice of both physician and provider and there is a general belief that a bigger hospital will provide them with better treatment. This movement of patients is not compensated by the HIIS. Some local hospitals claim that up to 30 per cent of patients go to other regions or to the Clinical Centre in Ljubljana for their treatment.

Health care delivery is very decentralized in Slovenia, following traditions that date back to the Austro-Hungarian organization of health communities. With few exceptions, the average maximum distance that any Slovene citizen has to travel to reach their GP is not more than 10km. The number of home visits is falling.[4] This is a result of two factors: people now expect more from a visit to a surgery, and have better physical access to health services at the primary level.

The distribution of hospitals is slightly different but the majority of the population has hospital services within a 25km range. The development of a more dynamic health care market together with the opening of borders within the EU will make health care services more freely available and choice will be greater. But focus group participants also had expectations of greater internal mobility and believed this should be available to all categories of patients when their conditions can be treated better in certain institutions than others. They saw this as a potentially very important way of influencing the system, by reducing waiting times and developing healthy competition between physicians and hospitals.

Performance rankings were not seen as so important and most patients would not seek such information. The professional competence of doctors and other health professionals was taken at face value. Waiting times did not matter that much when patients had an assurance that they would be seen by top professionals. Some patients felt that all physicians should be trained equally well, so that it should not matter which physician examined them. For those who expressed this view, it was important that the state guarantees standards through quality assurance and control.

NEW ROLES FOR THE CITIZEN

Strengthening patients' rights

Article 51 of the Slovene Constitution defines the right to health care as one of a citizen's basic rights.[14] The same article also states that no one can be forced to undergo treatment unless the law specifically prescribes it. The Law on Health Services in Article 47 states:

> Everyone has the right to choose a physician and provider of health care, to consult with specialists chosen by him/herself or to request a second opinion, to know their diagnosis and the types of treatment available. He/she has the right to give or

withdraw consent for any intervention, to be informed about the diagnostic and therapeutic methods and effects and to decline the proposed interventions; to see his/her medical files related to his/her health condition, unless the physician judges that it would have a damaging effect on the patient's condition, has the right to confidentiality, to demand a transfer to another health care institution, to complain to the relevant authorities if he/she thinks that not all effective means to treat them have been used or that ethical principles were breached, to be informed about the treatment costs and receive an explanation of the bill for health services and to receive compensation for inadequate treatment. For children under the age of 15, parents or carers are authorised to exercise these rights on their behalf.

Under this law, all citizens enjoy a fairly high level of rights, comparable to the most developed countries of Europe. The Ministry of Health and the Slovene Consumers' Association have published a booklet entitled *Patient Rights and Responsibilities* which is distributed to all health care providers free of charge and should be available to all patients.[15] However, many patients believe their rights are not sufficiently respected. According to the Slovene Consumers' Association, one of the most common offences is that physicians are reluctant to give patients access to their medical records.[16] Patients refuse to accept the argument that it is inappropriate for them to see some test results, arguing that they cannot decide on the right treatment if they don't understand their own condition.[17]

It is rather worrying that about 10 per cent of those surveyed believed that their personal data is not treated confidentially.[18] There has also been significant criticism of the law on health care databases adopted in July 2000. This determines the way personal and health data are collected and how access to this information is regulated. However, there is a fear that information may reach unauthorized people, as databases are as numerous as the institutions, providers and physicians who hold them. They are not managed by authorized persons under special supervision and are only loosely regulated. The sheer numbers affect data security and potential abuse of confidential data is a real concern.

The basic health care legislation defines the main principles and procedures of a complaint system for patients. Written complaints can be addressed to individual health professionals, or to a special complaints body of the Medical Chamber. Complaints can be made anonymously. If the investigation finds incriminating evidence

Table 6.1 The focus groups in the Slovene study

Group	No. of participants	Age	Sex	Location	Health status
1	8	25–34	Female	Ljubljana	Healthy
2	8	25–34	Male	Ljubljana	Healthy
3	8	30–49	Female	Ljubljana	Recent inpatient
4	8	30–49	Male	Maribor	Recent inpatient
5	8	35–49	Female	Ljubljana	Healthy
6	8	35–49	Male	Novo Mesto	Healthy
7	8	50–64	Female	Maribor	Chronic illness
8	6	50–64	Male	Koper	Chronic illness

against a doctor or dentist, the prosecutor of the Medical Chamber takes over the case and investigates further. In less serious cases of poor or unfair treatment, any citizen has the right to complain to a complaints' officer within the Ministry of Health. That officer is then authorized to seek additional information and to direct the complainant to the relevant authorities if they wish to take further action.

Participation in policy making

Not discussed.

FOCUS GROUPS

Eight focus groups were conducted in June 2001, details of which are shown in Table 6.1.

NOTES

1 Emergency Medical Care Project, Ministry of Health of the Republic of Slovenia, 1995–2000.
2 Slovene Public Opinion Survey (SPOS) (1999) *Opinions on Health and the Healthcare system.* Ljublijana: Faculty of Social Sciences, Institute of Social Sciences.
3 Health Sector Management Project Slovenia, http://sigov3.sigov.si/mz/ang.
4 Adamic, M. *et al.* (1999) *Health in Slovenia.* Ljubljana: Institute of Public Health of the Republic of Slovenia.

5 National Healthcare Providers' Database, maintained by the Institute of Public Health of the Republic of Slovenia.

6 Kersnik, J. and Ropret, T. (2002) Evaluation of patient satisfaction in family practice patients with diverse ethnic backgrounds, *Swiss Medical Weekly*, 132(9–10): 121–4.

7 Kersnik, J. (2000) An evaluation of patient satisfaction with family practice care in Slovenia, *International Journal for Quality in Healthcare*, 12(2): 143–7.

8 Patient satisfaction with family practice: comparing Europe and Slovenia (2000) *Zdravniski Vestnik*, 69(1): 5–10.

9 Kersnik, J., Bossman, P. and Svab, I. (1998) The patients' leading reasons for choosing a personal family physician, *Zdrav Var*, 37(5–6): 185–190.

10 Cufar, A. (2001) *Pharmacists' performance, experiences*, personal communication.

11 Alidzanovic, G., Primozic, S., Frankic, D. and Cufar, A. (2001) Evaluation of the attitudes to self-treatment and to OTC medications in the inhabitants of the Gorenjska region, in A. Cufar, M. Cvelbar, J. Dolinar, D. Frankic, G. Hladnik and S. Primozic (eds) *Self-treatment: Possibilities and Perspectives of Self-treatment, Symposium Proceedings: Brdo pri Kranju, 23 March*. Ljubljana: Slovensko Farmacevtsko Drustvo.

12 Gorjup, V. and Gersak, B. (1998) Second opinion – a new possibility for patients and physicians, *Isis*, 7(6): 27–8.

13 Health Insurance Institute of Slovenia (1998) *Recommendations and Conclusions of the First Evaluation Conference of the Health Insurance Card Project in the Posavje Region, 11–12 June*. Catez: Health Insurance Institute of Slovenia.

14 Constitution of the Republic of Slovenia (1991).

15 Slovene Consumers' Association (1998) *Patients' Rights and Responsibilities in Slovenia*. Ljubljana: Slovene Consumers' Association.

16 Flis, V. (1999) Medical records and patient rights, in J. Rebersek-Gorisek and V. Flis (eds) *Zbornik Medicina in pravo 1996, 1997, 1998*. Maribor: Splosna Bolnisnica Maribor.

17 Mekina, I. (2000) Orwell from the surgery, *Magazine Mladina*, 45.

18 Krasko, I. (1999) Patients are very sharp critics, *Newspaper Dnevnik*, 27 July.

7

SPAIN

OPINIONS ABOUT THE HEALTH CARE SYSTEM

The present system

Spain's highly decentralized health service means that models in each region vary. While some regions have their own health plans, it has not proved possible to institute an integrated national health plan, except in certain key areas. For these reasons the conclusions from research carried out in a specific geographical area cannot be reliably extrapolated to the whole Spanish health system.

Health care reform has taken place gradually throughout Spain, albeit unevenly. Two key elements in the reform programme were the establishment of stable teams of medical professionals working full-time in primary health care centres, and the building of new hospitals in rural areas to reverse the geographical inequalities generated during the Franco era. The aim was to promote equal access to health services by correcting structural inequalities. With the exception of certain regions like Catalonia, which has a mix of private and public funding, the main hospitals in Spain are owned by central or regional government and are university-affiliated and publicly funded.

The increasing life expectancy of the Spanish population has led to an increase in chronic diseases and in co-morbidities, creating new demands for the treatment of specific diseases such as oncology, geriatrics and mental health. Ageing and dependence are key issues on the agenda of the Spanish health authorities. In addition, other health needs are increasing, such as those related to unhealthy life-styles, the abuse of intravenous drugs, AIDS and traffic injuries.

Such problems have spawned the development of new public health programmes. These programmes, which focused initially on infectious diseases, have now been extended to cover the prevention of all diseases and the promotion of healthy lifestyles. Increasing migration from America, Africa and Eastern Europe has focused attention on the need to develop health care services that can address the health needs of minority groups.

Access and responsiveness

According to surveys conducted in the 1990s, Spaniards see health as the most important area of public investment. Most people were positive about the public health system, with 61 per cent saying it runs well or quite well, although many felt that certain changes were needed.[1] They were even more positive about GP care, with older people being most likely to express satisfaction. People with recent experience of health care were more likely to rate it highly than those who had not used it recently.

However, 61 per cent of respondents believed that investment in health care was insufficient, and 77 per cent felt it needed to be reorganized.[2] The fact that those people who enjoyed good health were more likely to call for additional investment was surprising.[3] Highest priority was given to increasing/improving the number of hospital beds (32 per cent), medical technology (22 per cent) and primary health care (20 per cent).[4] Paradoxically, few people would be willing to see increases in taxation to pay for health care.

In 1991, 72 per cent of Spaniards indicated that they were very or quite satisfied with health services used in the 12 months prior to the interview, whereas 28 per cent were dissatisfied.[2] The greatest dissatisfaction was found among the youngest respondents and those with higher salaries. Respondents were fairly satisfied with aspects related to the interaction between user and provider (how they were treated, explanations given and quality of visit), but were less satisfied with factors related to access (waiting time at home and in the doctor's office). When asked to comment on their own health centre, most people were satisfied with treatment by doctors and nursing staff, provision of information about their health problem, the appointments system and the location of the clinic. They were less happy about the length of time spent waiting at the centre. Very few respondents made complaints about inappropriate care.[5]

Access problems generated the greatest level of dissatisfaction and complaints in most of the studies reviewed. Patients want health centres to meet a set of basic demands, such as having efficient appointment systems, reducing or eradicating waiting lists for specialist care (and in certain areas even GP care), simplifying the bureaucracy of an organization which they deem is too bound up with red tape and reducing delays for non-urgent admissions to hospital. Better access arrangements were perceived to be one of the strongest features of the private sector, but private services are only available to those people who enjoy a higher level of income.

The proximity of primary health care centres is much appreciated in Spain and many patients prefer to visit their GP first rather than go straight to a specialist. A 1990 survey found that patients visited their doctors on average six times a year.[6] As far as emergencies are concerned, 19 per cent of those polled used these services in the 12 months before the interview. Of those, 75 per cent went without seeing a doctor first, and 60 per cent went to hospital emergency departments whereas 22 per cent visited non-hospital emergency services.[5] It is interesting to note that the use of hospital emergency services is determined by waiting times in regular care services, as well as by the distance to the health centre. Thus, visits to emergency rooms substitute for visits to GPs and specialists: a 10 per cent fall in the waiting time to access GPs was found to give rise to a 20 per cent fall in the use of emergency services.[7]

Focus group participants were concerned about heavy demand on doctors and long waiting times, although this seemed to be less of a problem in rural areas: *'They do not answer calls for a medical appointment and you have to go to the health centre and wait one hour to get an appointment'; 'If I am going to visit a doctor because I have flu, by the time I get an appointment I no longer have the flu'.*

This was also the most consistent complaint about specialist services, particularly when the condition involved some degree of pain. Participants felt that doctors and patients had different ideas about what constituted an emergency:

For elective surgery you can wait all your life: for me it is urgent, but I do not know if it is for the doctors.

I had endometrial cancer and in the public system I would have had to wait four months to be treated. I did not want to wait so long so I went through the private system and in four days I underwent surgery.

Emergency services were considered to be the most efficient way into the system. It was thought that anyone with a clinical condition had a better chance of good, fast care if they were admitted to an emergency ward: '*Specialists see you for a few minutes. If you go down in the middle of the street and the SAMUR [mobile emergency care] take you to an emergency room, then you get the scanner . . . then they do everything for you*'. However, long waiting times could be a problem here too: '*I, for example, can be in an emergency room in the public system and I can be in the waiting room for five hours, dying, vomiting on the floor, until I'm seen*'.

Structure and organization

Most of the population use the public health service when they have a health problem. The public system accounts for 85 per cent of primary health care visits, 71 per cent of specialized care visits, 88 per cent of hospital admissions and 90 per cent of emergency visits.[1] According to the National Health Survey of 1997, 85 per cent of the population went to a public centre in their last visit to the doctor, 7 per cent to a private centre and 6 per cent to a medical company.[8] For those who were hospitalised, 82 per cent of the total cost was paid by the government and 10 per cent by private health insurance.

Most Spaniards (71 per cent) are in favour of state-funded health care, while just over a quarter (26 per cent) defend the coexistence of public and private systems.[4] In a 1991 survey, 17 per cent of Spaniards said they had private health insurance and had used a private service in their last visit to the doctor.[2] The proportion using private health care has remained fairly constant throughout the last decade.

Cost and efficiency

Currently, co-payment is only required for drug prescriptions in primary health care, but the proposal to introduce more co-payments has given rise to widespread public opposition. People do not see it as an effective form of cost control and believe it should only be implemented for medicines and hospital accommodation costs. People in full employment pay 40 per cent of the cost of a prescription, with reductions for patients with specific chronic diseases. Some high-cost drugs are subsidized. User contributions or co-payments are supported by those in higher income groups, but 66 per cent of housewives did not agree with co-payments for medical prescriptions and 90 per cent felt there should be no co-payment for visits to the doctor or emergency room.[3,9]

Willingness to pay an additional amount as a means of cutting waiting times was considered acceptable by only 12 per cent of respondents in a study among people waiting for cataract surgery in the city of Barcelona.[10] Generally speaking, co-payment does not seem to be acceptable in Spain and currently politicians refuse to legislate for it.

Equity

Not discussed.

PATIENTS' VIEWS OF HEALTH PROFESSIONALS

Doctors

Focus group participants considered a personal and continuing relationship with a family doctor to be an important feature of a quality service. The possibility of consulting any available doctor in order to be seen quickly was only seen as attractive in the area of specialist care. Being able to get an appointment quickly was seen as a different type of benefit, not comparable to that of having your own doctor. Each consultation with a doctor was part of a process, not an isolated episode, and continuity of care was considered very important:

> *If you have a good doctor, nothing in the world makes you accept a change. First of all, he knows you, and how to treat you. We are talking about the doctor you see regularly, who knows your problems, who advises you.*

> *It depends whether it's specialist care or primary care. In primary care I prefer to wait and see the same doctor. It is better than jumping from one doctor to another, even if I have to wait. My doctor knows me, knows my medical record, asks me how I am, informs me about new drugs to lower blood cholesterol . . . The other doctor doesn't know me and he has to ask questions . . . They have changed my doctor recently and I am feeling very bad about it.*

However, continuity was only valued if the relationship with the doctor was a good one: '*What is clear is that if you get a doctor that you like and trust, and he provides solutions to your problems, then you are not going to change him. If you have a doctor who confronts you or doesn't treat you well, you might want to change'.*

Participants felt the heavy demand on doctors sometimes adversely affected the relationship, which could become impersonal and time-restricted. In these situations patients were not given adequate information about their condition and treatment. They were not examined and diagnostic tests were not requested. Routine prescription was the rule and there was a resistance to specialist referrals:

If I go with a problem, doctors pay no attention to it, irrespective of the type of problem. Maybe they see me as a young person or they feel that I am worrying about things unnecessarily.

For me, the experience is always negative. You go, they see you and check your health faster. I know there are queues, but they need a quick solution because demand is increasing.

The physician-patient relationship is inappropriate . . . they have half an hour to see 30 patients and, thus, they see 30 patients in half an hour.

Despite the fact that the health care system was regarded as inefficient, both specialists and surgeons were generally considered to be highly qualified professionals. The occasional mention of diagnostic or similar problems did not damage the essentially positive image of them:

I think there are good professionals in the public health care system, but there is a lack of manpower and good organization. The resources go first to the public system and, after that, to the private system. Thus, the public system has the best resources and professionals.

My experience was positive. They caught me in time. The cardiologist gave me an ECG and a stroke was detected. Thanks to his competence.

Focus group participants wanted health care in the future to be more personalized. They consistently expressed the desire for a personal relationship with their practitioner, in which mutual exchange of information takes place. Mutual trust was seen as more important than a prompt consultation with an unknown doctor. For serious clinical conditions, where there is no treatment available locally, they would like the possibility of consulting the best specialists elsewhere.

Nurses

The only available study indicates that patients prefer to receive treatment from their doctor than from a nurse. Thus, in the management of chronic conditions the majority of patients preferred the doctor (54 per cent), although 27 per cent did not care if it was the doctor or the nurse.[11] The nurse's role was clearly defined by patients. They were seen as a complement to doctors, providing supplementary information and reassuring the patient. They soften the medical setting and offer support in distressing situations. They are easier to talk to than doctors, are attentive and caring, and in closer contact with the patient than doctors.

Pharmacists

Apart from doctors, the patients in the focus groups also relied on pharmacists, who were considered to have an important role in health care. They were seen as playing a complementary role to that of doctors, having some information doctors may not have and giving better drug advice than doctors. However, it was also felt that their present role was the right one and that they should not be allowed to prescribe.

ALTERNATIVE WAYS OF ACCESSING HEALTH ADVICE

Telephone

Greater use of the telephone was considered potentially helpful by focus group participants for 'minor' consultations or for less serious diseases. It was also considered adequate for guidance on administrative issues. But for the diagnostic consultation, the telephone, like the internet, was viewed as impersonal and prone to risks or biases: *'A telephone consultation is better than the internet. You can talk with the person'; 'I prefer to see the doctor's face and be seen by him'*.

Telemedicine

The idea of consulting a doctor via a telephone and videolink (i.e. telemedicine) was viewed by participants in the same way as use of the internet or the phone. It was considered practical for some things, including minor conditions or health-related questions, but not for those consultations that require a real diagnosis. Once again, the main reservation was that it might replace the essential personal contact between doctor and patient: *'No, the treatment would not be personal, and if he has to check your pulse, how can he do that by phone or video?'; 'It is like sex without contact, I want physical contact. The more contact with a doctor, the better we are'*.

EXTENDING THE SCOPE OF MEDICAL CARE

Complementary therapies

In a 1991 survey, 6 per cent indicated that they regularly visit 'quack' doctors or healers (*curandero*).[2] Complementary therapies were seldom mentioned spontaneously in the focus groups, but occasionally they were seen as a valid complement to more conventional treatment. Homeopathy, acupuncture and natural medicine were mentioned. The arguments in favour of this type of therapy were mainly related to the problems that some patients had had with orthodox medicines and the supposed lower cost.

New medicines and biotechnologies

Spanish people's attitude to technological and scientific advances was addressed in a survey carried out by the Centro de Investigaciones Sociológicas.[12] This study revealed a wariness about the latest scientific breakthroughs in the fields of biotechnology and genetic engineering. Some 57 per cent of respondents considered that scientific progress in these areas was quite or very dangerous, and 60 per cent felt that scientific advances in the coming years would entail major risks. Overall, 38 per cent of the respondents felt that the risks of scientific and technological progress would outweigh the potential benefits. Despite this negative outlook, 52 per cent of Spaniards regarded the use of genetic tests for the diagnosis of hereditary diseases and for the development of new medical treatments as acceptable. Moreover, most respondents agreed with the use of new biotechnologies to cure serious diseases (83 per cent), to prevent children from inheriting serious genetic diseases (81 per cent), to reduce the risk of eventually suffering from serious diseases (73 per cent) or to prevent children from inheriting mild diseases (63 per cent).

Despite the fact that 72 per cent of respondents believed that human cloning would be possible in the near future, 73 per cent considered that the health authorities should do their utmost to prevent investigation and experiments in this field, and 81 per cent agreed with a specific law to prevent or forbid the cloning of human beings.

As genetic tests are not widely available at the moment, focus group participants tended to adopt a more theoretical attitude to these possibilities. On the positive side, if a predisposition to a disease were found, treatment could be offered to avoid its occurrence. They could also extend life expectancy. However, there was no sign that these patients would agree to take such tests. Some participants said they preferred not to know if they had a predisposition to a particular disease, but others would like to know if it could prevent illness or the possible transmission of a disease to their children:

> *The study of chromosomes is out there and it helps to prevent future diseases, it is a great advance.*

> *I am going to have children, yes, I would like to know.*

> *If you told a person that he is going to have a heart attack at 30 years it might affect him and he might have the attack at that moment due to psychological disturbance.*

> *If you feel good, you are good, and therefore you don't take any tests.*

One in four respondents to a 1991 survey said they did not have access to the most modern medical technology.[2] Medical innovations are widely disseminated through mass media reports, which might explain why those with a higher level of education complain that they have difficulty in accessing these new technologies.[13] These complaints were more pronounced among those who expressed greater dissatisfaction with the health services generally.

INFORMATION FOR PATIENTS

Health information needs

The exchange of high quality information can only take place in the context of a more equal doctor-patient relationship based on mutual trust. One of the aims of the development and modernization of primary health care services in Spain has been to improve doctor-patient communication, but these reforms have not yet reached all parts of Spain. The situation is made even more difficult when the patient sees different doctors for the same clinical condition.

Information about health and medicine is difficult to access in Spain, even for health professionals. Libraries with major collections tend to belong to large hospitals and universities. Digital libraries have yet to get off the ground and telecommunications vary across the country. There are major shortcomings in rural areas and primary health care centres. Nevertheless, coverage of health issues in the media has grown progressively. As the annual evaluation carried out by the Observatory of Scientific Communication of the Universitat Pompeu Fabra shows, the number of items about health published in 2000 (11,945) was almost twice the number published in 1997 (5984).[14]

Among focus group participants, the general attitude towards 'wanting to know' was diverse. Some hints of differences between men and women were apparent, regardless of the age and type of patient. Men seemed more inclined to ignore health-related topics, even those that might directly affect them. Women were more active in the search for information. People living in rural areas and younger people were less interested in health topics: *'I don't want to know anything, I don't want any information, I want a fast cure'.*

Patients with specific conditions expressed a range of attitudes from an explicit wish not to know about the disease, to passive acceptance and a lack of interest in information once available, to more active information-seeking. The demand for information was related, almost invariably, to a specific disease. It is significant that no other general health and prevention issues were mentioned.

Patients in the focus groups distinguished between information received from medical institutions and that provided by other sources. Information provided by a GP was part of a two-way process, in which the patient was particularly sensitive to personal advice given by the doctor. When information was not part of a good communication process, it caused dissatisfaction:

First what you expect is eye contact, that they hear you and, once you have explained your symptoms, he gives you satisfactory answers, prescribes you a treatment and orders regular check-ups.

When they give you information it should be understandable, because sometimes they begin to talk, and talk, and talk . . . and you think: well, he must have thought I was beside him when he was studying medicine!

Information sources

The most important information source in the opinion of all the groups was the family doctor: *'I do think the best source of information is to go to the doctor and tell him what's wrong. Leave the consultation knowing what you have and then you do not need to search for information'.*

Other sources of information were also mentioned, depending on specific needs. Pharmacists were seen as the most consistently satisfactory information source, second in importance after doctors. Libraries were thought to require a high level of motivation. They were used only in cases of specific, intense need: *'When my father had a heart problem, I went to a library to search for information. I also searched the internet'.*

Health care organizations were regarded as good starting points for information on health-related topics and specific conditions. Organizations such as social services, the Red Cross, organ donation or disability groups were highly valued for the information they provide. Scientific journals satisfied an interest in more obscure topics and the television programme *In Good Hands* was mentioned as an example of information not specifically sought after, but enticing enough to keep the audience interested.

Health websites

The number of internet users in Spain is estimated to be 20 per cent of the population with an uneven distribution depending on geographic location, ranging from more than 21 per cent in Catalonia to 9 per cent in Castilla, la Mancha and Galicia.[15] It seems evident that with a growing number of users (from 6 per cent to 20 per cent in one year), and access becoming more economical and straightforward, the internet will increasingly become a major source of free health information. This is confirmed by the current proliferation of websites targeting health users, some of them driven by major advertising campaigns, and the attempts by the government to develop websites to promote health information for the general public. The National Health Institute's strategic programme (INSALUD 2000) includes 'The INSALUD Telemedicine Plan' which aims to apply information technology to the management of health care in several fields: telemedicine (remote medical care including consultation, diagnosis, monitoring), patient management and administration, health information for the general public, and training and information for professionals. The future of the internet in Spanish health care will depend on whether the right technological investments are made, and on a cultural change that makes the use of technology such as internet access via television sets more widespread.

Focus group participants valued internet searches due to the great amount of information they generate, but they require some degree of motivation, or at least curiosity. They saw the internet as providing fast, immediate access to information. They felt it would dramatically change the information exchange between health providers and patients, but trust in its effectiveness varied depending on the type of service required. Thus, access to information on a particular disease was valued more highly than the possibility of a 'virtual' consultation with a doctor or specialist. This possibility raised both doubts and concern about errors and misinterpretation:

> *If doctors can commit errors in a face-to-face relationship, you can imagine what can happen with the internet! Well, if you have the flu, it might work, they can prescribe you Couldina* [a drug for flu] *and so on, but if it is for a serious clinical condition, it's a bit more difficult.*

> *I do not think the internet is very reliable, because you don't know who you are talking to. He can introduce himself as a doctor or something but . . . I do not see too much reliability.*

In order to avoid these risks it was felt that contact should only be with a doctor familiar with the patient's history, that only minor illnesses should be beated in this way and that there should be audio and video support. For older patients, the physical presence of the doctor was seen as essential. The main complaint was the coldness of the internet compared to the warmer doctor-patient contact in the surgery: '*I can check the internet for minor conditions and non-essential questions, but if it is for a major illness I need to see a doctor face-to-face and see how he uses the technology*'.

Other ways in which participants thought the internet might be useful included booking a medical appointment, choosing a specialist, requesting a prescription and for access to information on the performance of health professionals.

PATIENT EMPOWERMENT

Self-diagnosis, self-medication, self-care

The National Health Survey of 1997 indicated that most of the respondents received their drug prescriptions from their doctors.[8] Self-medication was only reported for minor complaints such as fever and flu and is limited by Spanish legislation, which restricts the dispensing of drugs without a doctor's prescription. Despite this, studies have been carried out in local settings that suggest an increase in bacterial resistance associated with self-medicated antibiotics.

Self-help groups have only recently emerged in Spain, and are highly developed in certain areas of the country, such as Navarra, and less so in others. Some groups, for people with diseases such as AIDS, cancer or multiple sclerosis, are professionally organized, while others depend on voluntary participation of patients or their relatives. There is an organization that represents health care professionals dealing with consumer requests (Sociedad Española de Atención al Usuario de la Sanidad – *The Spanish Society of Attention to Healthcare Consumers*) and, recently, a new umbrella organization, the State Confederation of Patients, has been created to represent patient groups. In spite of these organized efforts, the evolution of patients' rights has not kept pace with developments in other European countries and North America.

Focus group participants expressed a range of attitudes towards taking responsibility for their own health. Some were unwilling to take the most elementary measures, not just preventive steps, but also those related to their own condition, while others saw themselves as fully responsible for at least some aspects of their own health care. They visited the doctor whenever they felt ill, were active in their demand for information, wanted to be given a choice of treatments, had regular check-ups and played an active role in their relationship with the doctor: '*I disagree that we have to accept every doctor's order. It is not possible because sometimes they get it wrong. Sometimes you have to get a second opinion*'.

Others showed a lack of control over their own health care. They were reluctant to visit the practitioner, did not dare to request information or accepted partial and simplified medical explanations, did not have regular check-ups, were unconfident in their relationship with their doctor and ignored the effect of certain lifestyles on disease and its prevention: '*I am very passive. I wait until something happens*'; '*I had surgery and the doctor tried to explain the treatment to me. I did not understand anything and I told him: I trust you . . . don't tell me anything more. Prescribe what will cure me'.*

Involvement in treatment decisions

The relationship between doctors and patients in Spain continues to be paternalistic on the whole. This is reinforced by four main factors: the inheritance of a charismatic professional model, the public nature of the health services, the persistence of a model of democratic transition and poor access to health information, particularly by the elderly and in rural areas. A more equal doctor-patient relationship is expected to take root in urban settings, associated with the emergence of a more educated and informed user and a professional who is more willing to listen to patients. Concepts such as shared decision making, concordance or patient empowerment are new to the health system of Spain. The implementation of these ideas will depend to a large extent on the existence of health professionals who are better prepared to share decisions with their patients and on the establishment of patient organizations that promote mediation between health professionals, health managers and patients.

Most patients want to obtain clear and understandable information on their disease, its treatment and prognosis, from a doctor who is willing to clear up any doubts that arise and inform them openly about the consequences and side-effects of treatment choices. On the other hand, existing evidence suggests that patients do not rate active participation as a priority. Freedom to express their opinions, individual responsibility and shared decision making did not seem to be particularly important to Spanish patients, perhaps a result of the traditional paternalistic model of care that prevailed up until the last decade. Patients were not accustomed to participating in decisions affecting their health and consequently did not expect their doctors to encourage them to do so. However, in recent years younger patients have become more demanding and critical of the care they receive.

The concept of free choice is a recurring one in different election campaigns and is more developed in urban settings and in the areas of general medicine, gynaecology and paediatrics. Choice of treatment is not easily available in the Spanish health system and can only be exercised by the most informed patients. The introduction of a reference price system also limits the choice of pharmaceutical products.

Nevertheless, the changes that have impacted on the Spanish health system are giving rise to the appearance of a new type of health service user, who could be called the 'informed user'.[16] Traditionally, inequalities of knowledge between doctor and patient had a very specific influence on their respective roles. The gulf was widened by the belief that illness was a taboo subject, limited to the experts. The relationship was paternalistic, based on authority and experience. Rising educational standards and the information revolution have led to the emergence of a more informed user, keen to be more involved in decisions about treatment.

Electronic patient-held records

The introduction of the clinical record has increased patients' confidence in the health system, enabling them to find out more about their disease and its progress. The clinical record is theoretically the property of the patient but it is always held centrally, so it is not easy for the patient to access it.

There was unanimous support in the focus groups for the idea of an electronic card that could hold an individual's complete medical history. It was felt that patients would be able to carry this information with them all the time and health professionals would have quick access to it when needed. This was seen as particularly useful in the case of accidents or emergencies. It would be possible to keep the information permanently updated and connect it to a data bank. Errors, bureaucracy and loss of time could be avoided: *'You can go travelling, they have all the information. Allergies, operations . . . All the data that might be of interest for a doctor if something happens. Prescribed drugs . . . all this will be there'*. The only perceived disadvantage was the risk of loss of control over personal data and abuse of confidential information: *'The negative side would be if somebody steals it and knows its contents. It should be code protected. Something that guarantees privacy'*.

Choosing where to receive care

The potential for travelling around the country to access specialist health services is extensive, since high-technology hospitals are located in the big cities and major urban settings where very new technology is available. Innovative treatments, with a few exceptions, tend to be located in university hospitals that are mainly publicly funded. Access to treatments outside Spain is only possible in exceptional circumstances.

The evidence indicates that most patients want to be able to access the health care they need as close as possible to their homes. The close proximity of general medicine or paediatric services is an important satisfaction factor.[1] The importance of proximity implies that many people would be willing to forego a better quality of health care if they were forced to travel some distance to get it. In the only study we found in which patients were questioned about the possibility of travelling to get better health care, only 31 per cent of them were willing to travel to another town.[11] Regarding hospital care, 74 per cent said the closest hospital was less than 30 minutes away from their home.[2] Distance between home and hospital was related to socioeconomic status, with those in lower socioeconomic groups having to travel greater distances.

For focus group participants, willingness to travel depended on the type of clinical condition, the degree of severity and the treatments available. Patients tended to prefer to receive treatment in more familiar and easily accessible locations, except for extreme life-threatening conditions. There is an underlying need to feel safe and secure in times of illness: *'It is good because there are always centres more specialized in a specific problem. If you were burnt you could always go to the centre with more experience in treating burns instead of going to your local centre'; 'It's important that health care is closer to people not the contrary'.*

NEW ROLES FOR THE CITIZEN

Strengthening patients' rights

Articles 10 and 11 of the General Health Law of 1986 established the rights and obligations of patients. Subsequently, different regional governments have published reports that extend and develop these legal precepts.

Asked to discuss their rights as patients, the participants in the recent focus groups specifically mentioned *'The right to receive care within reasonable time'* and *'The right to be well attended'*, together with the right to request and receive information in understandable terms about one's disease and the alternative treatments available, and to make a decision based on the information received.

Issues of confidentiality and data protection are a novelty

in Spain, and are associated with the promotion of a national data protection law (LORTA) and with the controversy in Europe over the transmission of epidemiological data between databases. These issues were the subject of debate between professionals recently following the monitoring of HIV infection records from anonymous blood donors and the European directive on epidemiological data. But it should be emphasized that neither the general public nor health professionals have a great deal of training and expertise in matters related to confidentiality and privacy in Spain.

Participation in policy making

Priority-setting initiatives in the health system in Spain have not yet involved the public. The political debate is still limited to specialized forums of health experts. Although several attempts have been made to get people involved in decision-making in priority setting and the distribution of health resources, they have been limited to specific research related to cost-benefit analysis.[17] There is no tradition in Spanish politics of involving the public in health policy making.[18]

In 1995 a Ministry of Health and Consumption survey asked whether the health system provided the same services to everyone regardless of where they lived, their age, their social status and the seriousness of their disease. Although a majority answered yes in all categories, substantial minorities disagreed: 37 per cent felt that equity was affected by place of residence, 25 per cent by age, 31 per cent by social status and 36 per cent by the type of illness. There was also a direct relationship between perception of inequality and dissatisfaction with the health services used in the previous year.[3]

Spain may witness greater participation of consumers in health issues in the future. At the moment, with the exception of a few specific patient organizations and health user units (departments within primary care centres and hospitals dealing with patient concerns), consumers' interests are protected by the National Organization of Consumers and Users.

FOCUS GROUPS

Six focus groups were conducted in July 2001, details of which are shown in Table 7.1.

Table 7.1 The focus groups in the Spanish study

Group	No. of participants	Age	Sex	Location	Health status
1	9	18–30	Male/female	Madrid	Healthy
2	10	30–50	Male/female	Barcelona	Healthy
3	10	50–65	Male/female	Madrid	Chronic illness
4	9	50–65	Male/female	Barcelona	Chronic illness
5	7	30–50	Male/female	Alicante	Chronic illness
6	9	18–30	Male/female	Rural Castilla	Healthy

NOTES

1 Centro de Investigaciones Sociologicas (Centre for Sociological Investigations) (CIS), 1995.
2 Comision para le Evaluacion y Analisis del Sistema Nacional de Salud (Commission for the Evaluation and Analysis of the National Health System) (CEAS), 1991.
3 Jovell, A.J. (1994) Salud o sanidad: análisis sociológico de los servicios sanitarios. Tesis doctoral, Departamento de Sociología y Metodología de las Ciencias Sociales, Universidad de Barcelona.
4 Centro de Investigacion de la Realidad Social (Social Reality Investigation Centre) (CIRES), 1990.
5 Centro de Investigaciones Sociologicas (Centre for Sociological Investigations) (CIS), 1990.
6 Comision para le Evaluacion y Analisis del Sistema Nacional de Salud (Commission for the Evaluation and Analysis of the National Health System) (CEAS), 1990.
7 Puig-Junoy, J., Saez, M. and Martinez-Garcia, E. (1998) Why do patients prefer hospital emergency visits? A nested multinomial logit analysis for patient-initiated contacts, *Healthcare Management Science*, 1(1): 39–52.
8 Encuesta Nacional de Salud (National Health Survey) (ENS), 1997.
9 Confederacion Espanola de Organizaciones de Amas de Casa, Consumidores y Usuarios (Spanish Confederation of Organisations of Housewives, Consumers and Users) (CEACCU), 1996.
10 Dunn, E., Black, C., Alonso, J., Norregaard, J.C. and Anderson, G.F. (1997) Patients' acceptance of waiting for cataract surgery: what makes a wait too long? *Social Science and Medicine*, 44(11): 1603–10.
11 Lorente Arenas, F., García Villamil, P. and Castro Ortiz, E. (1998) Gestión moderna de una consulta de Atención Primaria. Valoración crítica de los usuarios, *Cent Salud*, 6(4): 242–8.
12 Centro de Investigaciones Sociologicas (Centre for Sociological Investigations) (CIS), 1997.

13 Jovell, A.J. (1993) Society and health: clinical epidemiology, health status assessment, and policy implications. Doctoral dissertation, School of Public Health, Harvard University.

14 Infome Quiral 2000 (2001) Observatorio de la Comunicación Científica y Médica, UPF. Barcelona: Fundación Privada Vila Casas.

15 Encuesta General de Medios (General Mass Media Survey) (EGM), May 2001.

16 Jovell, A.J. (1999) El usuario informado: ¿utopía, realidad o moda? *Atención al Usuario*, 1: 4–6.

17 Gaminde, I. (1999) Priorities in healthcare: a perspective from Spain, *Health Policy*, 50(1–2): 55–70.

18 Honigsbaum, F., Calltorp, J., Ham, C. and Holmström, S. (1995) *Priority Setting Processes for Healthcare*. Oxford: Radcliffe Medical Press.

8

SWEDEN

OPINIONS ABOUT THE HEALTH CARE SYSTEM

The present system

The Swedish health care system is a regionally based, publicly financed and, to a very high degree, publicly provided national health service. It is organized on three political levels: national, regional and local. The county councils at the regional level, together with central government, are the basis of the health care system. During the 1980s, responsibility for most health care planning was decentralized from the national level to the county councils. In 1992 responsibility for long-term inpatient care and social welfare services for the disabled and elderly was transferred from the county councils to the local municipalities. A few years later the municipalities took over additional responsibility for services for physically disabled people and for those suffering from long-term mental illnesses.

Access and responsiveness

A recent study showed that health services and universities are among the most trusted institutions in society.[1] Several studies during the 1990s revealed strong support for the Swedish public health care system.[1,2] More recently, however, shortages of resources and staff have become the focus of media attention and political debate. Access to primary care and to certain treatments has become more difficult.

Many focus group participants expressed the view that in comparison to other countries, Swedish health care is generally good and those who really need health care usually still get it: '*I think that Swedish health care is good, in an international perspective. A substantial part of the tax we pay is spent on keeping health services of high quality*'.

However, they also talked of difficulties in getting treatment in the public system with some patients being forced to turn to private clinics. Women with rheumatic disease mentioned increased waiting times and a lack of resources for time-consuming patients like the elderly. Some younger women complained that they had waited up to five weeks to speak to a doctor on the telephone. Others reported long queues and waiting times, particularly for emergency and specialist care: '*You're almost afraid to go the emergency room knowing that you will be sitting there*'.

Although there is great trust in health professionals, opinions become more negative when considering the more detailed aspects of health care. The number of complaints is steadily increasing and growing dissatisfaction has been noted in the surveys conducted by the Federation of Swedish County Councils (FCC).[3] This is particularly so in the youngest age group with several studies confirming a more negative attitude among the young.[4,5] On the other hand, younger people are more inclined to think that health care services are equitably distributed than older groups.[6]

In 1992, the ruling government introduced a 'health care guarantee', listing 12 tests and treatments. Anyone needing these was guaranteed health care within three months. Due to its ineffectiveness, the guarantee was abolished in 1997 and replaced by a general 'access guarantee' under which patients are guaranteed to see a physician within certain time limits.[7] Access to health care services is still a major problem in Sweden and political aims do not always fit with the available resources.

In 1999, the right to choose a GP was introduced in law. A similar right had been introduced in 1994 but was abolished shortly afterwards when the Social Democrats came into power. However, the shortage of physicians means that not all patients are able to exercise this right. In 1999, 2400 people living in Stockholm were asked about access to their GPs. About 25 per cent said they had to wait longer than was acceptable.[8] A similar result was found in a national study among 3200 Swedes the following year.[9] The number of people saying they had to wait an unacceptable length of time had almost doubled between 1994 and 1999.[10] During 1999 it was estimated that 30,000 patients in Stockholm county visited the hospitals' emergency departments because they could not get an appointment with their family doctor within a reasonable time.[11] Longer waiting times at primary health care centres and in telephone queues all over Sweden have made the access situation in primary health care one of the leading topics on the health policy agenda. Among those patients getting through, just 10 per cent were disappointed with the advice offered in their telephone contact.[12]

To improve information on waiting times, the Federation of County Councils launched a national website giving waiting times for various diagnoses at hospitals throughout Sweden. The aim was to make this information publicly available and to make it easier for patients to receive care at a hospital where the waiting time was shorter. However, the website has been criticized for 'guessing waiting times' and some have judged it as of no value to the general population.[13]

Among both decision makers and the general public, support for increasing health care resources has grown.[14] Focus group participants were afraid that there would be an increased shortage of qualified staff in the future due to reductions in staffing levels and low rates of pay, and that patients would be forced to pay more for medicines and tests. Some participants thought health care would get worse and patients would be forced to pay more through private insurance: *'If you are really ill, you won't be able to get insurance'.*

Structure and organization

There has been considerable debate about hospital closures and privatization of health services. Some small hospitals have been compelled to close, which has caused consternation and anger among local populations. In some areas, primary care services have been unified in medical centres, while in others attempts to centralize activities have failed. Shortage of health care personnel has also provoked discussion as commercial staffing agencies increase their market share. Provider-purchaser models attracted new political interest when a couple of public hospitals became private. In response the government introduced legislation to prevent further privatization of public hospitals.

The general public was asked about their attitude towards private hospitals in three different polls conducted during the same month. The results were conflicting. Depending on the wording of the questions, the share of positive answers varied from 30 per cent to 82 per cent.[15] This variation may be due to the fact that the number of private hospitals in Sweden is still very small, and few respondents were likely to have had any experience of them.

Focus group participants discussed the issue of privatization of parts of the service. Younger men had noticed an increase in the number of private clinics and some had followed the debates concerning privatization of parts of the health service: *'I have learned that health care is getting more and more privatized. It's probably okay for those who can afford it but I guess for the man on the street this development is not good. The result will be low quality health care for the rest of us'*.

Cost and efficiency

In one study, questions were asked about preferences for improving health care funding by increasing taxation, or by complementary private health care insurance or user charges.[14] Politicians and the public preferred increased taxes, but doctors advocated user fees and complementary insurance.[16] Private health care insurance is becoming more popular but it still plays a minor role in the Swedish financing system. Focus group participants did not want to have to pay more for health care in the future because they thought they were already paying enough, but they were afraid that the cost of private health insurance would increase.

One of the most pressing dilemmas concerns the steadily rising cost of drugs and the problem of so-called 'orphan drugs' – i.e. those aimed at patients with rare conditions. In an attempt to curb the increasing cost of pharmaceutical products, a drug reform programme was initiated in 1998 when the county councils took over responsibility for drug reimbursement from the state. This was intended to focus on the total drugs bill as well as the cost to the counties. In addition, the patients' share of the cost of drugs was increased under a reformed Drug Benefit Scheme. Methods to reduce public expenditure on drugs have been the subject of lively debate, particularly in the light of the demand for Viagra and Xenical. The reform programme was expected to be fully implemented by 2001, but has been delayed. The county councils will take over the majority of the responsibility for the public drug bill, and the tug-of-war between the national and the regional arenas has become the focus of much debate.

The strong influence of certain patient organizations makes it hard for politicians to control the introduction of new expensive pharmaceuticals targeted at large patient groups, even if the cost-efficiency ratio is low. Smaller patient groups are disadvantaged because of their minor importance as voters or consumers, but they still gain some public support. In an attitude survey, 70–80 per cent of surveyed pharmacists and physicians agreed fully or partly that drugs with only marginal effects should receive lower subsidies so that expensive medicines for patients with serious diseases can be provided instead.[17]

Several studies have tried to estimate the extent to which people choose not to buy prescribed medicines or consult a doctor because of the cost. The numbers vary in different studies, but the common tendency is for younger people to do so to a greater extent than older people.[18,19,20] About 3 per cent of the population refrains partly or wholly from medical consultations for financial reasons, and about 4 per cent say they try to avoid buying medicines on prescription,[21] but the seriousness of the health care needs in these situations is unknown.[22]

Despite opposition to increased patient fees or decreased subsidies for pharmaceuticals, a majority of people in one study thought that it was right that a patient should pay the whole cost if the physician prescribed a drug from which the patient was not expected to bene-fit.[17] Co-payments find support among the public, particularly when directed towards people with unhealthy lifestyles.[14] In most studies, one third of respondents were prepared to let smokers, drinkers or people who are overweight go to the back of the queue or pay extra. But there is strong resistance to the notion of allowing people who pay extra to get their treatment faster.[23]

Confidence in the welfare system and its ability to cope with future challenges seems to have collapsed over the last decade. The current system still has strong support, but three out of four citizens believe they will have to pay extra insurance or save money to guarantee themselves reasonable care in their old age.[24] Younger participants, in particular, were very aware of the financial crisis in the health service and the risk of having to pay for health services themselves: *'I believe that we will have to pay more if we are going to be able to afford health care today and tomorrow. It is getting more expensive with medication and treatments and I'm afraid that the citizens will have to pay it out of their own pockets'.*

Equity

Sweden has a political tradition of equity and different parts of the public health care system, including trade unions, provider organizations and political institutions, all have a role in striving to achieve this. Attention has been focused on equitable access for patients in different parts of the country,[25] access for men and women,[4] rich and poor,[26] old and young.[27] The argument that access to health care should not be restricted on grounds of ability to pay is a powerful one. It has been used in the debates on 'lifestyle' medicines and priority-setting in health care. The trade-off between the goal of equity and other goals such as health maximization or patients' freedom of choice is frequently discussed.

Health care debates during recent years have focused on the 'economic crisis' and the restoration of public finances. Different cost containment strategies have been introduced and criticized, and care of older people and long-term psychiatric patients has attracted particular attention. Neglected medical and social needs among these groups seem mainly to be a problem in the bigger cities but the picture is quite unclear, despite numerous official reports trying to estimate unmet needs and health differences.[25, 26, 28]

Focus group participants were afraid that those who are already socially excluded would be particularly disadvantaged in the future. It was felt that there should be more transparency about health care funding in order to guarantee that money is spent where it should be. Some participants were also anxious about the increasing demands placed on the health service by an ageing population.

The fact that some patients do not get the treatment considered necessary was of great concern to participants. Younger participants were concerned that shortages of staff would mean even less available time for patients and longer waiting times. They also expressed the concern that the national government appears to be withdrawing from health care management and that young people are being treated at the expense of elderly people: *'Young and old people should have the same rights'*. Some participants were afraid that Swedish health care was being 'Americanized': *'I expect health services to get worse, like in America, I'm sure I'll have to have my own health insurance and if you're already sick you won't be able to sign on. Society will split into two groups'*.

PATIENTS' VIEWS OF HEALTH PROFESSIONALS

Doctors

In a study among 1207 people in five Swedish counties, 76 per cent said they were pleased with their experiences of physicians over the years. The most positive respondents were those with longer health care experience.[17] Among primary care patients, 96 per cent reported positive experiences with the way they were treated by health care professionals and 92 per cent were satisfied with the medical competence of the staff.[5] Younger respondents tended to be more dissatisfied on both counts.

In a 1998 study carried out by the Swedish Institute for Health Economics, 1543 primary care patients were asked what they valued most when consulting a GP.[29] Good communication skills including friendliness, information-sharing and the doctor's knowledge of the patient's medical background were considered most important by all age groups. The only exception was respondents in the 18–40 age group, who valued participation in treatment decisions more than the doctor's knowledge of their medical history. Patients were also asked to agree or disagree with two statements regarding the quality of the physicians. Only 10 per cent of the respondents fully agreed with the statement '*The quality of Swedish GPs is so high on average that it doesn't matter who treats you*'. In the case of the second statement, '*The quality of Swedish hospital physicians is so high on average that it doesn't matter who treats you*', 20 per cent of the respondents agreed fully. Slightly less than half of the respondents partly agreed with both statements.

Female participants felt that doctors were under too much stress to spend time with their patients and consequently there was a lack of personal contact and individualized treatment. Insecurity arose from conflicting information supplied by different doctors, and participants felt they had to dig for information themselves: '*When you finally meet the doctor, you do not get the time that you feel is necessary for you*'.

Younger participants talked of the inconvenience of repeated tests when they move from one hospital to another or if specimens are lost, and of economy measures that make it more difficult for health professionals to fulfil their duties. They thought doctors should receive more training in psychology so they could offer a more holistic approach to health care.

In a study carried out in 1998, 4000 patients at eight hospitals were asked about their attitudes towards quality in health care services.[30] Although more than 80 per cent of the patients surveyed responded that they had confidence in the doctor who treated them, more than 40 per cent said they did not receive enough information on how the disease or its side-effects would affect routine living, and about a fifth of the patients (21 per cent) said they did not wholly understand the risks and benefits in relation to their treatment. In a survey conducted in 1999, respect was mentioned as the most important single factor in the health care consultation. Waiting times were not felt to be so important, but more opportunity to choose was mentioned by 65 per cent of the respondents.[31]

When asked about their confidence in different types of health professional, respondents in a large telephone survey said they preferred private GPs and district nurses, while public GPs received fewer votes.[3] The growing gap between needs and resources seems to be most manifest in the primary care sector and many complaints to local patient boards concern poor access and lack of patient information and dialogue.

Demand for services is higher among the elderly, who generally need to see a physician more frequently, often with diffuse symptoms and pre-existing diagnoses. Older respondents are particularly keen to establish a long-term relationship with a physician they deem reliable.[32] In a study including 4000 patients with diabetes, only 45 per cent of the respondents had been able to choose their own GP. Several patients complained about having to change doctor between each visit at the primary care centre, but thanks to the nurse they still felt some sense of continuity in their care and treatment.[33]

Focus group participants reacted negatively to the idea of reducing waiting time by seeing a different doctor. They felt that there is no time to provide a new doctor with all the necessary information relating to a long-standing condition. They would be forced to repeat the same information to different doctors, and there would be a higher risk of meeting a doctor who did not have the relevant skills: '*In the last five years, I've met new doctors each time I visited the hospital. And I tell you, it isn't fun having to tell the story of your life to a complete stranger who doesn't listen because he hasn't got the time*'.

Continuity of care was considered to be an important element of successful treatment. There was felt to be a risk that different doctors would offer contradictory medical advice, and that seeing different doctors all the time would increase the possibility of medical errors. Participants also felt less secure when meeting a new doctor who they did not know.

However, younger participants were prepared to see a different doctor for more minor conditions and some felt that the doctor-patient relationship was so impersonal already that they might as well see different doctors: '*It gives you a false sense of security if you only meet with one physician. I really don't think it matters. In my experience, the relationship between physician and patient is on a very formal level'.*

Nurses

The younger focus group participants had great confidence in nurses, but while the young women felt they should have more responsibility, the young men thought the existing balance of responsibility between doctors and nurses was about right. It was generally felt that nurses should only be given more responsibility if they have the necessary skills and patients feel comfortable about it. An important part of the nurse's work was to provide the patient with emotional support, but responsibility for prescribing medicines should stay with the doctor. Younger males also thought more male nurses might raise the status of the profession.

Pharmacists

Participants considered that pharmacists have sufficient responsibility. They strongly believed that patients should see a doctor if they want drugs on prescription.

ALTERNATIVE WAYS OF ACCESSING HEALTH ADVICE

Telephone

Most focus group participants thought the telephone could be a useful complement to personal contact as long as patients always have the opportunity to see their doctor face-to-face when necessary. Personal contact was felt to be essential for a correct diagnosis. The telephone was seen as most useful for quick access to information about less serious conditions: *'Calling your doctor is an alternative, particularly when the consultation concerns simple issues. However, when the problem is more complex, then you will probably need a physical visit'.*

Young male participants pointed out that the telephone demands good verbal skills, which could be a problem for some people, particularly the elderly. Some participants thought that greater telephone use was undesirable as all patients need face-to-face contact and a personal service from their doctor: *'I still believe that the human interaction is very important'.*

Telemedicine

Like the telephone, participants thought that telemedicine could be a useful complement to, but not a replacement for, face-to-face contact with a doctor: '*You need a human being who touches you*'. Younger participants thought telemedicine could be useful for those patients who lived a long way from the nearest doctor. Some also thought that GPs should have the opportunity of talking to specialists using a live telephone and videolink. This could enable patients to access specialist care more quickly and reduce waiting times. There was concern among some participants that it would be difficult for the elderly and the sick to handle the technology.

EXTENDING THE SCOPE OF MEDICAL CARE

Complementary therapies

The market for alternative therapies is steadily increasing, and natural remedies were sold for 1.6 billion Swedish crowns in 2000. One in ten Swedes uses natural cures daily and one in four uses alternative medicine at least once a year. In a study among primary care patients in 1998, 15 per cent reported using alternative medicine regularly and the well educated were slightly over-represented.[5]

Following legislation in 1993, complementary medicines have been classified into three groups: natural remedies that have been approved by the Pharmaceutical Department; free-listed natural remedies that await approval; and natural remedies that do not have any official status.[34] These medicines must be produced in accordance with good manufacturing practice and have been traditionally used or have proven beneficial effects.

Every second consumer has a positive, or very positive, attitude towards alternative drugs, while most physicians still hold a neutral or negative attitude.[35] Younger physicians have a more positive view.[36] Nurses generally show positive attitudes towards alternative therapies and drugs, and a majority of all health personnel in a Stockholm study of 1997 said that natural cures were useful complements to conventional medicine.[37] The strong interest among patients has led to a growing interest among health providers in learning more about these drugs.[38] Alternative treatments like homeopathy, chiropractic treatments and acupuncture are also gaining interest. It is estimated that 2.5 million Swedes use these treatments.[37]

Young participants in the focus groups had a very positive attitude to complementary therapies. They wanted to see greater cooperation between alternative and conventional medicine, but felt it was important that complementary medicine was well regulated in order to avoid charlatans.

New medicines and biotechnologies

In April 2001 the government took a sudden decision to cut the subsidies for diet and impotence drugs, except for certain patient groups. Sweden was one of very few countries where no limit on cost repayment had been placed on these drugs, and some sort of harmonization with the rest of Europe was reached. It was expected that the public would support this decision. In a survey commissioned by the official Prioritization Delegation, a majority of people, physicians, politicians and administrators thought these medicines should be subsidised 'sometimes' or 'never'.[38] Among the general public, and especially the young, more sympathy was expressed towards impotence drugs: one in three respondents aged 18–30 wanted impotence drugs to 'always' be subsidized.

INFORMATION FOR PATIENTS

Health information needs

One of the most recurrent results in Swedish patient surveys is the apparently insatiable hunger for information. Younger and better educated respondents are more willing to admit that they lack sufficient information – for example, on choosing a GP – and they express a greater demand for more information.[32] In a study, conducted among 1543 primary care patients, the same tendency was found.[5] Perceived information level was associated with better health status. Among respondents who regarded themselves as healthier than people of the same age, 57 per cent felt fully informed about their disease or medical problem, while only 37 per cent of those in poorer health felt fully informed.

There was a feeling among several focus group participants that patients had to seek out information themselves in order to take better control of their care: '*You have to be well enough to be sick so you can take care of yourself and ask the right kind of questions*'.

The type of information participants felt would be useful

included: information about self-care, new research, side-effects of medication, disease management, length of treatment, appropriate treatment and health status. Participants did not completely trust written information and were more confident about the information they received from family and friends, pharmacists or others with the same condition as themselves: *'You talk and you ask questions, for example about if you know a good doctor'; 'I pick up most information from other people'*.

In theory, participants felt that everyone should feel free to ask their doctor whatever questions they wanted to: *'There are no stupid questions'*. But participants with rheumatic disease felt that they held back from asking questions for fear of appearing stupid. They also thought that if they asked too many questions they might be forced to change their doctor. Younger female participants felt they never got answers to all their questions because there was never enough time. They often forgot to ask some questions and doctors used language they did not always understand. They believed that patients have to be firm and argue their case if they are to get the information they want: *'I never get any answers, but I don't give up. You want to know as much as possible'*.

Younger male participants often found it difficult to ask questions, owing to a sense of insecurity or inferiority in relation to the doctor, fear of appearing stupid, fear of the answer and the doctor's lack of interpersonal skills.

Information sources

In a study by Garpenby and Husberg, people's preferred sources of health information were evaluated.[26] The most preferred source was the doctor, followed by the family. Those least preferred were the internet and patient organizations. Similar results have been reported elsewhere.[17] The study also found that women used a significantly wider range of information sources than men, including alternative therapy books, pharmacists and other health professionals. Fallberg and Svanberg's study of 4000 patients with diabetes, showed that nurses specializing in diabetes were judged equal to physicians as preferred sources of information.[33]

Health websites

In 1999 the National Pharmacy in collaboration with a majority of Swedish counties established the Infomedica website (www.infomedica.se) to 'strengthen the role of citizens in the health service by offering access to reliable knowledge and information'. The site is interactive, allowing people to ask questions online to the GP in charge. In addition, most Swedish county councils have developed their own websites where they provide public information on patients' rights, the structure and organization of the health service and recent developments in the county. Most pharmaceutical companies also have websites with specific patient information.

In a study by the Centre for Technology Assessment (CMT), 48 per cent of the respondents said they had access to the internet and 11 per cent said they had used the internet to search for health-related information.[26] The study also showed that there is a strong relationship between age and access to the internet. Among respondents aged 18–29, 80 per cent of all males and 63 per cent of all females reported having access to the internet. The corresponding figures for respondents aged 65–74 were 12 per cent for males and 4 per cent for females.

In a study involving diabetic patients, only 10 per cent of respondents said they regarded the internet as an 'important' or 'very important' source of information.[33] Focus group participants' confidence in information found on the internet depended on the source. They were more likely to trust information provided by individual patients. Participants with chronic diseases, generally older patients, were much less likely to use the internet: *'I don't access the internet. I'm somewhat of an opponent to it'*.

PATIENT EMPOWERMENT

Self-diagnosis, self-medication, self-care

It is said that 90 per cent of all health care in Sweden is carried out in the home, without the aid of health care professionals.[39] The combined effect of a better educated, well-informed and health conscious generation, an extended supply of treatments and drugs oriented towards quality of life, coupled with public resource problems, leads towards the increased practice of self-diagnosis, self-medication and use of over-the-counter medicines.

Some focus group participants felt that their only responsibility as patients was to keep appointments or cancel them as soon as possible if they could not keep them. Others thought they were also responsible for taking prescribed medicines, adopting a healthy lifestyle, talking over treatment decisions with doctors, doing what they could to control a disease and giving the doctor all the necessary information. Participants thought that giving patients the opportunity to carry out tests on their own might facilitate early diagnosis and that more information about the factors that aid recovery might help to bring about behavioural changes: *'The individual must have an understanding in order to be prepared to make sacrifices'*.

Involvement in treatment decisions

Under the Medical Health Services Act, Swedish health professionals are required to provide health services in agreement with the patient, and with concern and respect for their needs and wishes. This statement has been criticized for being too vague, both in terms of guiding health professionals on how to involve patients, but also in facilitating patients' participation. An official committee was asked to review the legislation. Their report, *The Patient is Right*,[40] concluded that due to the growing number of treatment options and variations in risk/benefit analysis, it is becoming more important to involve users in clinical decision making. From 1999 a new provision was added to the Medical Health Services Act under which clinical practitioners are required to let the patient choose when two or more treatment options are available. However, the obligation to let the patient choose is limited to alternatives within what is clinically accepted as 'scientific and proven knowledge' and there has to be a reasonable cost/benefit ratio.

The same provision also included the obligation to give patients the right to a second opinion if certain conditions prevail. This right only applies to patients with a life-threatening disease or a particularly critical illness. The National Board of Health and Welfare evaluated the reform of second opinion legislation in March 2000. The evaluation showed that nearly 90 per cent of clinicians had not experienced any changes as a result of the reform. It was also noted that the opportunity to seek a second opinion existed long before it became statutory. Indeed the new provision rather restricted the option.

In several studies, communication skills have been valued as the most important quality dimension, especially among young people.[4,32] It has been suggested that these skills are the easiest for patients to judge, but calls for dialogue, listening and information seem to be a sign of their greater self-confidence and desire for greater participation. Older people feel more strongly about being able to choose a doctor, while younger and well-educated individuals feel more strongly about the choice of treatment.[10] Most patients want physicians to inform them about the treatment options and their probable outcomes, and then decide which alternative to choose, either alone or in consultation with the physician.[5]

Focus group participants felt it was the responsibility of the health professional to carry out tests for disease, offer a diagnosis and a range of alternative treatments, prescribe the correct medication and provide information on the effects of that medication. They also thought that patients should be allowed to see the bill for their treatment so that they know how the money is being spent.

In general, participants felt patients exercise little control over their own health care. For example, they have no influence over when an examination is carried out and how long they might have to wait at the emergency reception. Younger female participants experienced 'a total lack of control' and participants generally wanted a greater say in their treatment. It was felt that those who paid had more control. Participants with rheumatic disease also thought they were sometimes criticized when they took responsibility for their own rehabilitation through massage and travel to a warmer climate: *'You get the feeling that they think this kind of treatment is a sort of luxury rehabilitation'.*

Some participants felt they lost control when they had to take advantage of personal contacts or resort to anger in order to receive necessary health care. Being obstinate and stubborn did not make participants feel good about themselves and they were afraid of being seen as a difficult patient.

Electronic patient-held records

Focus group participants liked the idea of carrying their medical history on a smart card as long as there was a system in place that guaranteed information could not be abused. They saw a number of advantages, including quick access to the patient's medical history, increased efficiency (particularly in an emergency situation) and a reduction in the amount of paperwork in the health system. Moreover, patients would not need to repeat information to different doctors and important information would not be forgotten: *'If you are going to hospital after an accident and have a smart card they will know right away what kind of medication you need'.*

Younger male participants saw a potential risk in unauthorized access to sensitive material – for example, treatment for venereal disease: *'The negative thing is individual integrity. I mean, if your doctor can see in your medical file that you were infected with chlamydia some 20 years ago'.*

Choosing where to receive care

Most patients receive health care in their home county. With some limitations, patients are free to seek health care in other counties too. Sometimes this option is connected to the home county's inability to guarantee access within a certain time. But few patients seek health care in other counties, with the exception of people living in county border areas where the closest provider might be in the neighbouring county. The home county then has to pay this external provider according to a national schedule of rates. These are relatively advantageous to the providers and patients from other counties are welcome visitors.

Employees with private health care insurance might be forced to travel further to get their treatment quicker and the option to seek providers outside the home district or county council mainly attracts the better-off socioeconomic groups. Choosing to travel for treatment might be dictated by the time gains or the higher quality care expected.

In spite of the lively debate about free choice of health care provider in the EU, not many patients have tried this option. Many governments, including the Swedish, are reluctant to lose cost control if people seek expensive alternatives abroad. The rules regulating the public reimbursement system are not clear. The most well known examples of patients going abroad to receive their treatment are patients travelling to the UK for heart transplants. In the border area between Norway and Sweden some people cross the border when seeking care, and in southern Sweden increasing traffic between Denmark and Sweden is expected as a result of the new bridge bringing the two countries together. Some agreements between Swedish and Danish health care providers have already been signed.

Fifty national quality registers support clinicians and medical authorities in Sweden. Originally local research registers established in the 1970s, they have been gradually transformed into permanent national specialist registers administered by the National Board of Health and Welfare (SoS) and the Federation of County Councils (FCC). A majority of clinics participate and regularly publish new data. Those clinics that do not participate have been shown to have poorer results.[41] Some years ago SoS published mortality rates among patients with heart attacks admitted to different hospitals in Sweden, but criticism about the accuracy of the data (mostly from clinics with poor results) was harsh and questions were raised about whether the general public is able to understand and use outcomes data from hospitals. Since then there have been no more attempts to publish this kind of data.

Some focus group participants felt that sufficient performance information was available already. Others thought that for a number of reasons it was problematic. Doctors are learning new things all the time and mistakes can often be due to overwork and stress: '*If I'm ill, I would like to know if my doctor has made a mistake, which probably would make me choose another doctor. But thinking about health services today, I guess physicians don't make mistakes because of incompetence but because they are working under stress and have been working for 24 hours and all that'*.

Participants felt that performance measurement should be the responsibility of health professionals; patients should not have to worry whether doctors have the necessary skills. People do not want to be overloaded with information when they are ill and information about medical errors could lead to anxiety. Patients are unlikely to invest a lot of time and money in seeking a more qualified doctor anyway – it is waiting times that influence care-seeking behaviour. Clinics with the best record might start to charge extra. Participants were concerned about doctors' underperformance: '*I guess it is easier to feel confidence in someone, a doctor, performing well as a professional. But then again, there will be other doctors unemployed, due to incompetence and lack of trust on the part of the patients'*.

Others were reluctant to have performance indicators without the right to choose a specialist: '*It is not often that you are allowed to choose your own doctor. If you were referred to one that you knew was responsible for a terrible mistake, you would be dead scared'*.

However, the young male participants saw some advantages to making performance information more readily available. Doctors would gain confidence, knowing that they have performed well and there would be an increased opportunity for the patient to seek out the best health care.

NEW ROLES FOR THE CITIZEN

Strengthening patients' rights

In 1997 the government produced a report on patients' rights. In spite of the seductive title, *The Patient is Right*,[40] this report (and the later constitutional changes) did not contain any absolute rights, but rather widened the providers' obligations to guarantee a free choice of GP, access to individual information, choice of treatment alternative and the option to seek a second opinion for severely ill patients. The report said that this was because of the problems involved in defining patients' rights.

Access to medical records is one of the few absolute rights in Swedish health care legislation. Health professionals are obliged to present the medical record without any delay and are not allowed to ask why the patient wants to access their medical file. Patients are entitled not only to read their medical files, but also to have copies made and to have errors corrected, and any discriminating or disrespectful comments erased. If the practitioner refuses to let the patient read their file, or access is delayed without explanation, the patient can turn to the Regional Office of the National Board of Health and Welfare or to the Administrative County Court (Länsrätt). There are two exceptions to this principle. The first relates to the risk of jeopardizing the patient's recovery if access is granted, and the second relates to psychiatric patients, when the information provider risks being threatened or injured if the patient has access to the information.

Only health professionals directly involved in the care and treatment of the patient are allowed access to their medical records. In a recent case involving the care and treatment of a member of the Cabinet, a great number of health professionals were found to have accessed his medical file. Of these, 26 professionals were found by the Criminal Court not to be directly involved in his care. The case is still pending but in the first instance they were found guilty of breaking the rules of confidentiality and sentenced to pay a fine.

Focus group participants generally felt that patients had a right to health care when they needed it, to confidentiality and to information about their illness. In practice, they were often unaware of the right to a second opinion or to be treated with dignity and respect. Some participants thought there was a lack of information about patient rights because health professionals had little time to provide it. They felt that no one should be given a diagnosis without their permission. The complex issue of rights to treatment for lifestyle indications, (e.g. non-clinical obesity) was discussed. Participants felt that although patients have a right to treatment, they must also take responsibility for their own health.

There was a feeling that it was sometimes necessary to fight for your rights to health care. People who do not stand up for themselves are often treated as non-priority cases and end up at the back of the queue. Participants thought that this situation had worsened over the last ten years.

The National Board of Health and Welfare is the authority responsible for the safety of patients in all public and private health services. Since 1937 Swedish legislation has required all health institutions to file reports on any patient injury believed to be caused by a mistake or error.[42] This information is linked to an SoS database which collates all reported incidents nationally. However, due to the risk of being disciplined, the number of unreported incidents is estimated to be very high.[43] The SoS can report incidents to the Health Services Responsibility Board (HSAN), which in turn may impose sanctions, or revoke a licence to work as a health care professional. Patients can also complain directly to the HSAN. The information is then fed back to the health services to help prevent future incidents. Compensation for medical errors is arranged through the 'no fault' patient insurance schemes.

In a survey of 2200 surgical and orthopaedic patients from nine hospitals in the greater Stockholm area, more than 10 per cent of patients thought they had received the wrong treatment.[44] Another study among former patients found that every fourth person in the age group 18–34 felt disappointed with their health care consultation.[4] Among the changes participants in the focus groups wanted to see was reduced working time for doctors to reduce the risk of medical errors.

Participation in policy making

The gap between health needs and resources is growing in Sweden and prioritization is increasingly necessary. The 1997 parliamentary resolution on priority-setting in health care reflected the central ideas from the National Priorities Commission Report *Priorities in health care*.[45] The recommendations were formulated as general guidelines and the three ethical principles of human dignity, need and solidarity, and cost efficiency were laid down. Four groups of clinical examples, ranked in accordance with the ethical principles, serve as a tool for clinical and administrative personnel when setting priorities. The Swedish approach is comparatively general in design, a deliberate concession to clinical freedom.

The Swedish Parliamentary Priorities Commission invited public discussion on the conclusions of its final report. In several counties a large number of study circles met to discuss both *Priorities in health care* and *The Patient is Right*. The most common form of public input was through negotiations between politicians and patient representatives. Direct dialogue with patients is not usual in the counties, with some minor exceptions. Younger and well-educated individuals generally make greater demands for participation and influence than older people.[32] Studies have shown that younger people in Sweden are less ignorant, less bounded by authority and less willing to be manipulated than older generations.[46]

At the Swedish Institute for Health Economics, a number of surveys on the priority-setting theme have been conducted since 1993 to find out if people share health providers' views on the scarcity of health care resources and the need for rationing. A large number of people agreed fully or partly (92 per cent) with the statement that public health care should always offer the best possible care, irrespective of cost.[14] Among physicians the share was just 59 per cent. Another statement asserted that every individual should have their health care needs met, even if the problem is trivial. Some 40 per cent of people agreed fully, but among administrators and physicians the figures were just 5 and 6 per cent respectively. In an earlier study, 71 per cent of the primary care patients surveyed agreed fully with this proposition. The expectations of patients and the public seem to go far beyond those of the decision makers and exceed available health care resources.

However, in the Eurobarometer survey of 1998, almost half of the Swedes felt that limits should be set in public health care and some treatments should be given priority.[47] Compared to the answers from the six other European countries in the study, the Swedes were more inclined to use age as a legitimate criterion. The respondents from Sweden and the UK were also more positive towards meeting the need for increased funding with higher taxation (27 per cent). The recommendations in the two reports *Priorities in Healthcare* and *The Patient is Right* illustrated the potential conflicts between priority-setting and patient power. Patient demands are growing louder at the same time as the need for central planning is greater than ever.

Young and well-educated individuals generally make greater demands for participation and influence than older people.[32] This increased self-confidence among the young creates certain problems in a traditional social democratic society like Sweden. The common welfare policy has in some sense been a victim of its own success. One of its earlier aims was to create strong and competent citizens, but these empowered citizens came to embrace values and preferences ill at ease with the underlying welfare policy.[48] This does not mean that egalitarianism has come to an end, but rather changed its focus. The main concerns today may not be the distribution of food, clothing and shelter, as they were a century ago, but in the distribution of less tangible assets – what economists call 'knowledge capital'.[49]

Others have claimed that Swedish society, in spite of its collectivist rhetoric, has a history of manifest individualism.[50] Typical of the Swedish welfare system is the direct link between the individual and the state, and the subsidies and the laws that are directed towards the individual, not the family or community. The relatively minor importance of the family, the community, the church etc. makes the individual citizen more dependent on the public welfare system. The debates about future policy directions are therefore polarized between tax-financed collectivism or individualistic market solutions.

FOCUS GROUPS

Four focus group discussions were conducted in December 2001, details of which are shown in Table 8.1.

Table 8.1 The focus groups in the Swedish study

Group	No. of participants	Age	Sex	Location	Health status
1	5	24–63	Male/female	Borås	Diabetes
2	6	41–73	Female	Borås	Rheumatic disease
3	4	24–28	Female	Halmstad	Recent inpatient
4	5	19–25	Male	Halmstad	Recent inpatient

156   *The European patient of the future*

NOTES

1 Holmberg, S. and Weibull, L. (eds) (2000) *The New Society*. Göteborg: Göteborgs Universitet.
2 Svallfors, S. (1996), Klass, kön och välfärdsstatlig integration: om attityder till välfärdspolitiken, in J. Palme, and I. Wennemo (eds) *Generell välfärd. Hot och möjligheter?* Stockholm: Välfärdsprojektets skriftserie Fakta/Kunskap.
3 Landstingsförbundet (2001) *Vårdbarometern* (National Gallup survey). Stockholm: Federation of City Councils.
4 SOU (1996) *Jämställd vård. Olika vård på lika villkor*. Huvudbetänkande från Utredningen om bemötande av kvinnor och män inom hälso- och sjukvården. Stockholm: Socialdepartementet.
5 Rosén, P., Anell, A. and Hjortsberg, C. (2001) Patient views on choice and participation in primary health care, *Health Policy*, 55: 121–8.
6 Landstingsförbundet (1994) *Svenska folkets erfarenheter av och inställning till hälso-och sjukvården 1994*. Stockholm: Landstings-förbundet.
7 Anell, A., Persson, M. and Svensson, M. (1999) En behandlingsgaranti i sjukvården? Arbetsrapport no. 3. Lund: Institute for Health Economics.
8 Sorsaa, R. and Carlstedt, A. (2000) *Vad tycker du om sjukvården? Befolkningens syn på och erfarenheter av vården*, Vårdvärdering nr. 19. Stockholm: Inregia.
9 Landstingsförbundet (2000) *Tre av fyra får tid på vårdcentral inom en vecka*. Stockholm: Landstingsförbundet.
10 Genell-Andrén, K. (1994) *Vad tycker du om sjukvården?* Vårdvärdering. Stockholm: Inregia.
11 *Dagens Medicin* (2000) Petienter Klagar på låg tillgänglighet hos läkare, 16 May.
12 *Dagens Medicin* (2000) December: 18.
13 Karlberg, I. (2001) Vem är intresserad av gissade väntetider på nätet? *Landstingsvärlden*, 3.
14 Rosén, P. and Jansson, S. (2000) Attityder till vården, *Enkätstudie bland medborgare, politiker, administratörer och läkare om attityder till prioriteringar i vården*. Stockholm: Prioriteringsdelegationen.
15 *Dagens Nyheter*, Ar S:t Göran sämre än S:t Bure? 13 November.
16 Välfärdsföretagen (1999) *Välfärdstjänster och dess finansiering*. www.valfard.nu.
17 Rosén, P., Jansson, S. and Jendteg, S. (2000) *Subvention av läkemedel på recept – Vad tycker allmänhet, läkare och apotekspersonal?* Lund: Institute for Health Economics.
18 Socialstyrelsen (1997) *Folkhälsorapport*. Stockholm: Socialstyrelsen.
19 Socialstyrelsen (2000) *Patientavgifter och vårdefterfrågan. En kunskaps-översikt*. Stockholm: Socialstyrelsen.
20 SOU (2000) *Välfärd vid vägskälet, Delbetänkande från Kommittén Välfärdsbokslut*. Stockholm: Socialdepartementet.

21 SCB (2001) *200 000 tvingas avstå från vård.* Välfärdsbulletinen. Stockholm: Socialstyrelsen.
22 Jones, I. and Britten, N. (1998) Why do some patients not cash their prescriptions? *British Journal of General Practice*, 48: 903–5.
23 *Landstingsvärlden* (2000) Fler bör betala för vården, 31.
24 SIFO (1996) *Framtidens sjukvård* (news bulletin).
25 SOU (1998) *Tre städer – En storstadspolitik för hela landet.* Slutbetänkande av Storstadskommittén. Stockholm: Socialdepartementet.
26 CMT Rapport (2000) Hälsoinformation idag och i morgon. Östgötarnas användning av och förtroende för olika informationskällor. Linköping: CMT.
27 SOU (2000) *Välfärd, vård och omsorg.* Forskarvolym från Kommittén Välfärdsbokslut. Stockholm: Socialdepartementet.
28 SOU (2000) *Hälsa på lika villkor – nationella mål för folkhälsan.* Slutbetänkande från Nationella Folkhälsokommittén. Stockholm: Socialdepartementet.
29 Rosén, P., Anell, A., Hjortsberg, C. and Håkansson, A. (1998) *Patientpreferenser i primärvården – en empirisk undersökning kring patientinflytande*, Report no. 3. Lund: IHE.
30 Höglund, E. (1998) *Vad tycker patienten om vården?* Spri rapport 470. Stockholm: SPRI.
31 Vårdförbundet (1999) *Respekt viktigare än korta väntetider. Ny SIFO-undersökning om allmänhetens syn på sjukvården.* Stockholm: Vårdförbundet.
32 Anell, A., Rosén, P. and Hjortsberg, C. (1997) Choice and participation in the health services: a survey of preferences among Swedish residents, *Health Policy*, 40: 157–68.
33 Fallberg, L. and Svanberg, K. (2000) *We Evaluate our Healthcare: How Patients with Diabetes Value Quality in Health Services*, Delrapport 2. Gothenburg: Nordic School of Public Health.
34 *Farmaceutisk Revy*, Var tionde svensk nyttjar dagligen naturläkemedel och det blir bara fler, May 2000.
35 *Landstingsvärlden*, Populära naturmedel påverkar den vanliga vården, November 2000.
36 *Dagens Medicin* (1998) 2.
37 *Dagens Medicin* (1997) Vårdpersonal positiv till alternativmedicin, 21.
38 *Svenska Dagbladet* (1999) Den nya vården.
39 *Sydsvenska Dagbladet* (1997) Alternativmedicin ska bli rumsren, 23 September.
40 SOU (1997) *Patienten har rätt.* Stockholm: Socialdepartementet.
41 *Dagens Medicin* (1998) 8 December.
42 Ödegård, S. (1995) *Lex Maria – From Punishment to Prevention? A Study of Incident Reports to the SoS between 1989–1993.* Gothenburg: Nordic School of Public Health.
43 Riksdagens Revisorer (1994) *Disciplinary Actions in the Health Service.* Stockholm: Riksdagens Revisorer.

44 Bäckström, C., Carlstedt, A. *et al.* (1999) *Vad tycker du om sjukvården?* Vårdvärdering nr. 20. Allmänkirurgi, Ortopedi. Stockholm: Inregia.
45 SOU (1995) *Vårdens svåra val, Slutbetänkande från Prioriteringsutredningen.* Stockholm: Socialdepartementet.
46 Petterson, T. and Puranen, B. (2001) *The Nineties Report.* Stockholm: Institutet för Framtidsstudier.
47 Mossialos, E. and King, D. (1999) Citizens and rationing: analysis of a European survey, *Health Policy,* 49: 75–135.
48 Pettersson, T. and Geyer, K (1992) *Värderingsförändringar i Sverige.* Stockholm: Brevskolan.
49 Fogel, R.W. (2000) *The Fourth Great Awakening & the Future of Egalitarianism.* Chicago: University of Chicago Press.
50 SOU (1998) Bemäktiga individerna. Om domstolarna, lagen och de individuella rättigheterna i Sverige. Stockholm: Demokratiutredningens skrift nr 20 (Trägårdh, L). Stockholm: Socialdepartementet.

9

SWITZERLAND

OPINIONS ABOUT THE HEALTHCARE SYSTEM

The present system

In Switzerland, health care is mainly delivered by physicians in private practice (solo practice is still the most common model) and public hospitals where both inpatient and outpatient care is offered. In 1996, a long awaited revision of the federal law on sickness insurance came into effect. Besides formalizing the principle of universality, the law encourages more competition between the Swiss sickness funds, as one of several measures aimed at containing costs. The law specifies that only care that is effective, appropriate and efficient should be reimbursed in the framework of the statutory health care insurance. In addition, measures to assure quality of care should be agreed between health care providers and insurers.

There is an acknowledgement that the system must adapt to take account of the needs of an increasing number of patients of non-Swiss origin (19 per cent nationally, up to 43 per cent in Geneva). Steps are already being taken in this direction – for instance, more regular use of interpreters and mediators and measures to encourage health care professionals to be more sensitive to cultural differences. Other changes are also proposed, such as the development of services dedicated to teenagers[1] and paediatric services that allow parents a bigger role.[2] Specialist services are being set up, including clinics for pain relief, back problems, urinary incontinence, addiction and sporting injuries.

The Zurich Manifesto for health reform recommends limiting the supply of health care providers by reducing the numbers of medical students and jobs for physicians and cutting the number of transplant centres.[3] Such changes may involve greater travel and less choice for patients in the long term, but their impact is uncertain and there has been no research on how the public would react. The recommendation for more national coordination includes measures to improve cooperation between the federal and cantonal governments, but more radically also involves creating health care regions that would break down political cantonal boundaries into more meaningful health care units.

In 2000, the Federal Office for Social Insurance (OFAS) sponsored a representative population survey to assess public attitudes to the impact of the federal law on health insurance.[4] When asked to rate the current law on a scale of 1 to 10, people gave the system 7.25 for guaranteeing good medical care, 6.5 for providing sufficient care, 5.2 for adaptation to the needs of the population, 4.75 for fairness, 4.1 for affordability and 3.4 for cost containment. These results were echoed in another survey which found that 58 per cent of the population was satisfied with the health care system.[5] Furthermore, over 50 per cent believed that the quality of health care in Switzerland is better than anywhere else[6] and half of all respondents were content with the current services.[4]

This view was reflected among the focus group participants where the consensus was that the Swiss health care system is well organized and of high quality, especially when compared to those in other countries. The following strengths were listed: universal coverage, wide range of services included in basic health insurance, good access to hospitals and free choice of doctors. In addition, the French-speaking groups attributed the quality of the system to technology and to the skills of the health care professionals: *'Switzerland is a privileged country with an impressive range of care options and technology'*.

But the qualitative research also revealed concerns about the increasing complexity of the health care system. Participants who had undergone a negative experience often mentioned problems of organization or continuity of care, and the importance of adequate information allowing immediate referral to the right health professional was frequently highlighted.

Although the elderly population is healthier than before,[7] an ageing population combined with advances in the treatment of acute conditions will add to the burden of chronic conditions that must be addressed by the health service. Patients' expectations are changing as more people become aware of existing health services and of their rights as patients. There is a growing demand for more personalized health care.[8] The traditionally rather long hospital stays have been getting progressively shorter, leading to the development of day surgery clinics and home care. People seem to have a very positive view of these options.[9]

In 1995, 70 experts examined how the health care system would change in ten years.[10] An increasingly health conscious population, greater use of prevention, additional measures to improve patient safety, increased patient rights and a larger role for independent patient organizations were all envisaged.

In the French-speaking focus groups, the predominant expectation was a clear deterioration in the situation due to the centralization of certain health care activities, and the drive towards maximum efficiency and profitability. The German-speaking Swiss were more optimistic, citing a greater role for alternative medicine, expansion of preventive activities and more interdisciplinary collaboration as developments for the future.

Access and responsiveness

The Swiss health care system has been preoccupied with cost management and quality assessment. Patient satisfaction surveys and quality indicators are used by many Swiss hospitals in monitoring quality.[11] However, there is currently no standard patient satisfaction survey instrument, and since the objective is self-monitoring, the results of patient satisfaction surveys are not usually made public. Some hospitals have published their results, however. The surveys conducted at the University Hospital of Lausanne show that global satisfaction of inpatients has remained high (90 per cent) and stable between 1996 and 1999.[12] The nationwide network of hospitals found that 15 per cent of hospitals introducing changes following patient surveys cited improvements in patient satisfaction.[11]

Overall results from a study of 1027 patients comparing satisfaction levels in four different ambulatory care sites in Geneva indicate a moderate satisfaction with access, with lower satisfaction ratings for patients enrolled in a managed health care group (67 per cent) and patients visiting university clinics (66 per cent) compared to patients visiting private group practices (72 per cent).[13] A study among 1540 patients seen by 36 GPs found a high level of satisfaction with getting appointments (91 per cent), with receiving fast attention for urgent health problems (90 per cent) and with getting through to the practice on the phone (89 per cent). The study revealed lower satisfaction rates with physicians' phone availability (77 per cent) and the general waiting time (78 per cent).[14]

Structure and organization

The 1996 reforms officially authorized new models of care such as Health Maintenance Organisations (HMOs) although they had actually been in existence since 1990. An HMO is a type of plan that controls health care expenses by making cost-saving arrangements with physicians, hospitals and other health care providers. Currently, only 7 per cent of the Swiss population is registered in a managed care system and health care is mainly delivered by physicians in individual private practices.[15] Indeed, the economic incentive for people to change has been considered insufficient, and many individuals are attached to the traditional system.[13,16] Nevertheless, managed care is making inroads and the circumstances under which it is established and the extent to which choice remains a possibility are major considerations.[13]

The centrality of trust in family doctors was voiced repeatedly in the focus groups and represented the standard against which alternatives were judged. For instance, participants in the Swiss-German focus groups felt they would only be attracted to the HMO-type model if several doctors (e.g. GPs, specialists and physicians trained in alternative medicine) worked collaboratively to improve the quality of health care.

Cost and efficiency

One of the main features of the Swiss health care system is its high cost, the highest in Europe, amounting to more than 10 per cent of the GDP in 1999 and an average of more than €3500 per inhabitant per year.[17] Health care coverage is available to everyone in the country through a system of statutory, compulsory affiliation to a sickness fund for basic coverage.[18]

The most commonly used model of insurance allows open access to a primary or secondary care physician for the patient who has to pay a 10 per cent contribution to ambulatory care and an annual fee of €100. Premiums are fixed independently of income. In addition, complementary insurance can be purchased that allows access to private hospitals and to private sections of public hospitals. Medical expenses greater than the limit allowed within statutory sickness insurance may be reimbursed by complementary coverage. Moreover, additional medical care may be obtained that is not included in the basic package but is approved at the federal level.[19]

While the public seems to give the health system relatively good marks for quality, the high cost of health care is less popular. Insurance premiums have been rising more quickly than most individual incomes or the GDP.[20] One problem with high costs is that any proposal to ration health care is perceived unfavourably because people are reluctant to consider giving up services.[21]

The general view among health experts appears to be that since compulsory sickness insurance is so comprehensive, access is simply not a problem.[21] A public opinion survey in the Romandie (French-speaking area) found that few people forego a medical visit for financial reasons.[6]

In principle, access to health care is possible for everyone; people with financial difficulties receive support to help pay insurance premiums. But many focus group participants expressed concern about the development of a *'two-tier health care system'* based on the type of insurance held by the patient. Some participants emphasized the importance of guaranteeing access to basic care: *'Without basic care, we would be dead at 45'*.

For about ten years, discussions went on between the Swiss Medical Association and the sickness funds and insurance companies about a new medical tariff. One aim was to correct the discrepancy between 'overpaid' medical procedures and 'underpaid' services such as patient consultations. A new tariff was introduced in 2002.

Focus group participants were particularly concerned about the continually rising cost of insurance premiums. In French-speaking Switzerland, health insurance companies were generally regarded as very powerful organizations, mainly interested in safeguarding their own economic interests. In German-speaking Switzerland, the discussion focused on cost-driving factors such as wasteful practices by doctors and hospitals, high patient demand and excessive use of expensive technologies.

A high density of general and specialist physicians and a growing demand from patients are some explanations for the high and increasing volume of medical care.[22] Some Swiss-German focus group participants strongly believed there were too many doctors: *'There are so many doctors! Someone has to pay for all that, and that's where the costs are'*. Many also talked about the important role of patients themselves and the need to develop incentives to reduce demand on the health services.

In contrast to the focus groups in the German-speaking areas of Switzerland, groups in the Romandie frequently considered that there were too few health care professionals working in hospitals and other health care units. The excessive workload they carried as a consequence caused several problems and meant that not enough time was given to the patient in general: *'They don't always have the time to do everything as they would like to'*.

All focus group participants were resigned to continued increases in health insurance premiums and costs: *'Of course the costs are going to rise. We are already looking forward to the next increase in premiums'*.

Equity

Some focus group members thought that the Swiss health insurance system was discriminatory. The premiums paid are not related to income, leaving many women and families at a disadvantage. Private insurance was also considered too costly for the elderly, who often have to switch back to basic insurance in old age. Finally, some insurers do not pay the service providers' bills directly but reimburse the patients after they have paid the bills themselves, restricting access to care for people who have limited financial resources: *'The system is relatively discriminatory. There are two levels: wealthy people who can afford a very high level of coverage and others who do not enjoy the same privileges. I think everyone should have the same privileges'*.

Up to fivefold variations in the average health care cost per inhabitant per year have been observed between the cantons.[7] Apart from cultural differences, these differences are due to different health care policies between the cantons. People in the German-speaking region of the country are less likely to have additional insurance cover, particularly private, than people in the other parts of the country.[4] While hospital costs are shared equally between cantons and sickness funds, 90 per cent of ambulatory costs are paid by the sickness funds.

PATIENTS' VIEWS OF HEALTH PROFESSIONALS

Doctors

In a representative telephone survey of the general population conducted in 1997 (N = 2024), 46 per cent of the respondents observed that doctors had, sometimes or often, little time to listen to patients or to provide information.[23] A European comparison indicates discrepancies in both the medical and psychosocial aspects of communication with GPs in Switzerland.[24] Swiss patients reported the highest discrepancies between expectations and experiences (important/not performed) in relation to explanations of the likely prognosis (18 per cent), information about the seriousness of the problem (16 per cent) and the cause of symptoms (12 per cent). An additional concern was lack of explanation of test results (16 per cent).

Several focus groups in both regions criticized doctors and specialists for having too little time for the patient. In French-speaking Switzerland, participants further criticized doctors for not listening properly and highlighted the problems of communication between patient and doctor:

> *It's tough when one is a foreigner and doesn't speak easily. One doesn't understand well and can't say the things well.*

> *Well, OK for being more in charge . . . but doctors should learn better how to listen to patients. One gets a diagnosis but no time has been taken to listen to us. Before doing more prevention, they should first learn how to listen to the patient.*

A study in the Romandie shows that patients expect to be seen by the same physician when a follow-up visit is needed, indicating that continuity of care is very important (80 per cent).[25] Focus group participants were asked if they would be prepared to sacrifice continuity of care for more rapid appointments. In German-speaking Switzerland, this scenario reminded some participants of the HMO model, which few people had experienced first-hand. Others were reminded of medical interns, where there is lack of familiarity and no continuity. People felt that such models are fundamentally flawed: the focus appears to be on the disease rather than the patient, they offer inadequate or no follow-up treatment and would require patients to repeat the same information over and over to different doctors.

All participants stressed the importance of trust in the doctor-patient relationship. In Switzerland, many patients have established a long-term relationship with a GP. Even among the younger age groups, this relationship seemed indispensable: '*It's important to have a doctor who knows you and tracks your health. You have to have trust, not someone who imposes a doctor X or Y on you*'.

The majority of participants would only accept seeing a different doctor for minor health problems or emergencies. Participants wanted to be able to determine when they change doctors and which doctor they see in cases of serious illness.

Nurses

There is less information available on attitudes towards other health professionals, but a study in German-speaking Switzerland suggested that most patients still perceive nurses in their traditional role as carers and do not expect much technical expertise from them.[26] However, this study at the main hospital in Bern showed that patient satisfaction with nursing staff was related to their team spirit and that in turn was positively influenced by the presence of a specialist nurse.

With the exception of some older men, Swiss-German focus group participants were open to an increase in responsibilities for nurses. They recognized that nurses are more experienced than doctors in certain things and closer to patients. Prescribing over-the-counter medications would not be a problem, and more responsibilities could be envisaged if they received more training.

The suggestion that nurses should have a greater role was not well received in the French-speaking part of Switzerland. The main obstacles mentioned were their lack of training and the professional stress they already face, given their present workload. However, most participants were ready to accept an enlargement in their numbers and responsibilities providing they received appropriate training for their new tasks: *'If they were relieved somewhat of current duties and they receive further training, then yes'*.

Pharmacists

In recent years, there has been considerable debate about the way in which medicines are dispensed in Switzerland. A national survey showed that 60 per cent of respondents obtained their medicines mainly or exclusively from pharmacies and 40 per cent from physicians, with significant differences between French- and German-speaking Switzerland.[27] People who considered the provision of expert advice important (41 per cent) were more likely to get their medicine from their doctor, whereas people who considered friendliness more important (19 per cent) were more likely to do so from a pharmacy. Overall, 96 per cent were satisfied with their source of medication, but the study showed that doctors were much more likely than pharmacists to explain how to take the drugs, the effects of non-compliance and side-effects. Focus group participants in the Romandie clearly thought of pharmacists as salespeople and the suggestion that they should play a larger role was not well received: *'No, I wouldn't trust him because I see him more as a shopkeeper'.*

In the Swiss-German groups, some people were wary of pharmacists' qualifications, whereas others saw them as being highly qualified. While there was a recognition that people already get medications for minor ailments directly from the pharmacist, participants felt that diagnosis should remain with doctors. As in Romandie, conflict of interest was also the primary concern here. Some people in German-speaking Switzerland were uncomfortable about doctors prescribing and selling medications due to conflicts of interest: *'He who sells should not prescribe, and he who prescribes should not sell'.*

ALTERNATIVE WAYS OF ACCESSING HEALTH ADVICE

Telephone

The increased use of the telephone for long-distance consultations upset the majority of participants in the focus groups. Even though increased accessibility was viewed positively, the anonymity of these systems was felt to be unsettling, giving rise to mistrust. The importance of face-to-face contact, direct observation and hands-on examination were mentioned many times as fundamentals of medical practice. Participants felt it would be problematic to shift responsibility to the patients to describe their problems via these channels: *'Personally, I'm opposed to this system because I think that communication is very important. I know that if I go to the doctor's office, I can talk, and that already does me a lot of good'.*

A telephone helpline was considered potentially useful for minor problems or a chronic disease where the condition was already clear. It was also more acceptable if people could call their own doctor. However, people clearly drew the line there. A helpline was not considered appropriate for more serious conditions where trust is essential.

Telemedicine

Telemedicine and remote diagnostics are still primarily only discussed by professionals. Some health professionals consider telemedicine a promising tool for accessing expert opinion about a case without the need for the patient to travel.[28]

Some focus group participants reacted very strongly against tele-medicine, but others noted benefits for rural communities or as a means for medical experts to communicate with each other. At most, participants could accept telemedicine as 'long-distance counselling' but not as 'long-distance treatment'. The visual aspect of video could not replace a live consultation and people were unimpressed by the 'digital doctor's' qualifications. Several groups voiced their concern that such technologies would certainly drive up costs, at least in the short term: *'Even if he had extraordinary qualifications, I still need to be able to actually see my doctor'.*

EXTENDING THE SCOPE OF MEDICAL CARE

Complementary therapies

The role of complementary medicine is officially acknowledged in Switzerland and several therapies are reimbursed by insurance if delivered by a formally trained physician. OFAS is currently examining how to evaluate the clinical effectiveness, appropriateness and cost-effectiveness of complementary therapies and which criteria should be used to include a therapy in the basic package of compulsory sickness insurance. Alternative therapy courses have been introduced in the five schools of medicine, but it seems unlikely that they will eliminate the divergence between conventional and alternative forms of medicine.[29]

A national survey in 1995–6 found that 40 per cent of the population had used complementary medicine in the past 12 months, and 10 per cent consulted an alternative practitioner.[30] A cantonal survey conducted in Vaud in 2000 showed that a quarter of the population sample had consulted an alternative practitioner in the past 12 months.[31] Taken together, these figures suggest that the use of alternative medicine will continue to increase in Switzerland.

The typical profile of an alternative therapy user in Switzerland is female, aged 30–50, well educated, of Swiss nationality, and German-speaking.[30, 32] Only a small minority (6–20 per cent) use alternative therapies on the recommendation of their physician. Most users report greater scepticism of conventional medicine but still tend to see alternative therapies as a complement rather than a substitute.

All the focus groups in the German-speaking part of Switzerland voiced enthusiastic support for alternative medicine: *'I know a lot of people who have used alternative medicine, and it works well and costs less'*. In the French-speaking part, only women signalled acceptance of a greater role for alternative medicine. Although young French-speaking men showed some acceptance, it was only as a last resort or an additional option. Men aged 50 to 65 years indicated little interest: *'Why not if I have already tried everything before? But not as the first step. Not sceptical about homeopathy but not in the first place'*.

Overall, a large number of the participants had already had experience with alternative medicine. Moreover, Swiss-Germans and women in the Romandie believed that alternative medicine should receive greater recognition and become more accessible. Many participants expressed a strong desire for a closer collaboration between alternative and conventional medicine in general: *'It would be fruitful if traditional and alternative medicines could work together better'*.

New medicines and biotechnologies

New diagnostic and therapeutic health care technologies are usually available relatively quickly in Switzerland and are frequently introduced before formal acceptance for reimbursement. For example, a 'Network for Cancer Predisposition Testing and Counselling' was established in 1999 to advise physicians and patients on the complex issues of genetic testing and cancer.[33]

Some focus group participants saw the expected growth in health care technology as detrimental to personal contact. Others, especially some Swiss-German men, thought it would help to cut costs. In the French-speaking groups, not a single positive comment was recorded about genetic tests. Participants felt tests to measure the risk of falling ill would be going too far, would be too expensive and probably useless in the sense that these tests would not result in any changes in patients' behaviour.

In the Swiss-German groups, men were more receptive to genetic tests than women. Most men in one group agreed that self-testing was a matter of individual responsibility – for example, the early detection of disease. There was general agreement among the men in another group that they would use such tests if symptoms were already present. However, in the absence of symptoms, many could not imagine people being motivated to take such tests despite the benefits of early detection. Swiss-German women rejected the use of such tests, believing that personal responsibility should be developed

in other ways. Participants in both regions believed that this technology was potentially dangerous because it would make people
anxious about their state of health: *'I want prevention, but I don't
want to know that I will have cancer in five years'*.

INFORMATION FOR PATIENTS

Health information needs

A study in Zurich showed that provision of health information was
one of two main areas that patients felt needed improvement.[34]
Similar findings have been obtained in satisfaction surveys among
inpatients in the French-speaking part of the country.[12] In a survey
among the general adult population in the canton of Vaud, half
of the respondents reported having searched actively for health
information in the previous 12 months.[31] Three quarters of the
respondents said they could find the information they needed easily,
18 per cent said they found the information with difficulty and
7 per cent could not find any useful information. About half the
respondents said they would like to be able to use a free helpline or
special information centre.

Information sources

In addition to general media and health magazines, many cantonal
offices and insurance companies provide regular information for
patients. However, there is little data available on the use of, and
satisfaction with, such sources of information. These materials
tend to reinforce the idea of the physician as the key source of
information.

Focus group participants spontaneously cited a large number of
information sources on health. The most popular included books,
friends, family physicians, the internet, TV, pharmacists and newspaper articles. However, should health problems arise, the primary
source of information for the French-speaking groups was the doctor. Pharmacists, homeopaths and other health care professionals
and the internet were also mentioned: *'. . . medical books as well. But
patients already have a hard time to get a medical book . . . if I'm sick,
it's my doctor that I'm looking for'*.

GPs and pharmacists enjoyed the highest level of trust, whereas
trust in the internet was low. Even so, seeking detailed information

about health topics remains the province of more educated patients and was generally restricted to obtaining information on a particular problem. The specialized press and the mass media were important means of disseminating information, but participants were keenly aware that there is wide variation in the quality and trustworthiness of the information available.

Health websites

The population survey in the canton of Vaud asked which media people preferred for general health information.[31] The internet met with lower enthusiasm than traditional media: 35 per cent rejected the internet, compared to 23 per cent who rejected brochures, 24 per cent a telephone helpline and 13 per cent a visit to a health centre. While internet use was reported in all focus groups, most participants complained about information overload and having to wade through lots of irrelevant or conflicting information. Internet use was generally considered difficult for those with little or no experience. Even avid internet users stressed the need for a trustworthy gateway for health websites and regular quality control: *'If you land on the homepage of the Swiss Federal Office of Public Health, you know it's good, but there are 1000 sites'.*

PATIENT EMPOWERMENT

Self-diagnosis, self-medication, self-care

There was broad consensus amongst focus group participants that people should take on more responsibility for their own health. They believed that people should adopt a more balanced diet, minimize risk behaviours and exercise regularly. Besides staying healthy, the Swiss-Germans, in particular, thought people should also use health services more prudently – for example, using fewer and cheaper services. People also believed that the health care system should support people in taking responsibility. There should be more health education and incentives to assist people in making more economical choices. Participants under 30 years of age confessed to not knowing much about the health care system. Although people consulted various sources of information on health and did many things on their own before going to the doctor, they were clearly opposed to any suggestion that responsibility should be transferred from the professionals to the patient: *'It is not that easy to take responsibility for oneself. You have to learn and understand how'.*

Self-medication is common in Switzerland, where 26 per cent of available drugs are available without prescription.[35] Self-medication is practised by about 40 per cent of individuals and rates of use increase with age.[36]

There are over 2000 self-help groups in Switzerland covering some 300 different conditions and problems. Besides a national body named KOSCH, an organization exists in most cantons to help direct the public to local groups. The self-help groups have a combined total of 22,000 active members, and the national body dealt with 8000 inquiries in 1999 alone.

Involvement in treatment decisions

There have been several campaigns in Switzerland to promote patient empowerment in health care. However, the evaluation of one such campaign in Ticino concluded that only 7 per cent of doctors had noticed patients exercising their rights and in general there was no apparent impact on the doctor-patient relationship.[37] A recent study found that 60 per cent to 70 per cent of Swiss-Italian patients have a paternalistic relationship with their doctors.[5] A telephone survey among a representative sample of the Swiss population showed that nearly 90 per cent of respondents agreed that the doctor should take an authoritative role in treatment decision making, but over 90 per cent also agreed that the physician should make suggestions, leaving the final decision to the patient.[38] People using alternative medicines and younger people were less likely to approve an authoritative role for their doctor. In another representative telephone survey conducted in 1997 (N = 2024), 64 per cent of the respondents indicated that at the end of a consultation the decision was shared between the patient and the physician, whereas in 26 per cent of patients the decision was made by the physician.[23]

A study among patients consulting GPs revealed a low level of satisfaction (52 per cent) with the extent to which doctors take account of their preferences.[14] Only 37 per cent of inpatients said they had been given a choice regarding examination or treatment.[12] Patients in Zurich indicated that shared decision making in diagnosis and treatment was one of two main areas needing improvement.[34] A study in the Romandie showed that GPs rarely take into account patients' expectations, even when aware of them.[39]

Studies have shown that offering more information to patients on the efficacy of certain treatments might result in a decrease in demand. In the Ticino, the information campaign on hysterectomy led to a 30 per cent decrease in the number of operations.[40] Experts therefore stress the benefits of patient empowerment as a strategy for a more rational use of health care. Choice of treatment appears to be more a communication than a medical issue in Switzerland. People want more information about therapeutic choices, and this is one clear weak-spot in doctor-patient relationships. In Vaud, only 65 per cent of patients said they received information from their doctors on other treatment possibilities.[31] Indeed, people may be looking for other options on their own, as the use of alternative therapies would suggest.

Electronic patient-held records

In the future, an electronic or smart card containing the patient's medical history could replace the paper and electronic records presently used. This concept elicited different reactions from the focus group participants. Some found the idea promising whereas others found it dehumanizing: '*This doesn't help create a human link with your doctor. No one will pay any attention any more to anything but the card*'.

The advantages were pretty clear: convenient storage of important patient information that could be accessed by health care providers. This file could even be expanded to include visual data such as radiological imaging, saving costs between physicians and hospitals. As all information would be stored on the card, the patient would not have to worry about forgetting anything important. It would also save patients and physicians from repeating medical histories on admission. It would help to alleviate difficulties faced by patients who had a poor command of the local language. Importantly, the card could contribute to saving lives in emergencies or chronic illness.

Most participants could very well envisage this technology in practice but their acceptance would be largely determined by how it is set up. They felt strongly that the use of such cards should be voluntary, and patients should have the right to determine what kind of information is included on the card. Participants were particularly concerned about risks of misuse – for example, the unauthorized use of data by employers or health insurance companies, as well as the implications for medical confidentiality: '*What does a doctor need to know? What constitutes privacy?*'

Choosing where to receive care

Whereas freedom to choose a primary care physician, a health plan or a specialist does exist in the framework of compulsory sickness insurance, the choice of elective hospital care is limited to the canton where the person lives. The cost of health care delivered outside the canton of residence is paid by that canton, providing preliminary approval has been given. Complementary insurance offered by private insurance companies usually covers this care.

Due to the nature and complexity of the Swiss health care system and because Switzerland does not belong to the EU, opportunities to travel outside the country to obtain health care are limited. However, because drugs and medical devices are relatively expensive, some people do purchase over-the-counter drugs and eyewear (glasses, contact lenses) abroad. Some people also go abroad for dental care, which is not covered by the statutory sickness insurance.

In the focus groups there was a generally ambivalent attitude towards the possibility of greater access to performance information provided by health professionals and hospitals. Even though most participants welcomed greater transparency, they felt uneasy about what they would do with performance information. Many participants were afraid of being overwhelmed by such information. Most said they would prefer to get expert advice from an information centre or their own doctor. This type of information was considered useful for health professionals, but not necessarily for patients themselves: *'As a sick person, I'm not in a position to determine who's best. A doctor is more likely to know'*.

Participants questioned the definition of quality contained in performance indicators. Since quality criteria could be defined by the institutions themselves, they might not correspond to patients' own criteria. Several participants said that their appreciation of quality was based mainly on the time and attention given by the doctor during the consultation, and they felt the technical aspects of care, while certainly important, are secondary to the quality of the doctor-patient relationship.

Some participants also expressed a fear that making this information available would lead to more *'medical tourism'*, driving costs up even further. German-speaking Swiss expressed the concern that the fees of good doctors would rise as demand for them increased. However, some participants believed that performance information would assist patients in taking greater responsibility for their own health: *'In general, people are poorly informed about the health care system, so such a development, where you could see who charges how much for what, would be good'.*

NEW ROLES FOR THE CITIZEN

Strengthening patients' rights

Several cantonal health departments (e.g. Geneva and Ticino) and various patient organizations have launched campaigns to educate the general public about their rights as patients. They emphasize information, informed consent, access to patient records, rights to a second opinion and access to health care as guaranteed by federal laws. The few data collected to date suggest insufficient knowledge and little exercise of patients' rights in Switzerland, even though the Swiss consider principles such as self-determination important. However, over the last decade or so there has been a dramatic change in cantonal legislation on patients' rights.[41]

Under Swiss law, patients have the right to access and photocopy their medical records.[42] Furthermore, physicians are obliged to respect medical confidentiality that may only be lifted in the case of epidemics or with the patient's consent. However, in practice, medical records can be difficult to obtain, incomplete or useless.[43]

According to a public opinion survey,[6] over 80 per cent of the general population in the Romandie believe that absolute confidentiality is necessary to be able to discuss all matters with their physician. However, the first representative general population survey in Vaud showed that while 97 per cent of the respondents were familiar with medical confidentiality, 17 per cent thought that this meant that *physicians* could refuse to give information to the *patient*.[31] Furthermore, half believed that medical confidentiality meant physicians could share medical information with patients' relatives and health insurance agencies without patient consent. The authors conclude that current knowledge and exercise of patient's rights in this area is too vague.

In a study of patient satisfaction with GPs, patients expressed a relatively high level of satisfaction with the confidential treatment of personal data (83 per cent).[14] Similar satisfaction rates with the maintenance of confidentiality by hospital personnel have been observed (84 per cent in 1998 and 82 per cent in 1999).[12]

OFAS has recently indicated that, based on external data, the number of deaths per year due to medical error could be in the range of 2–3000. A public opinion survey suggested that the Swiss would like to make doctors accountable in cases of medical error.[6] The media has been the driver of this debate, and several expert forums are being organized. In addition, a national task force has recently been created to examine the whole question of medical errors and how to deal with them.[44]

The Swiss Patients Organisation handled 3570 queries in 2000, 44 per cent concerning physicians.[45] Serious disputes are generally referred to the dedicated office at the Swiss Medical Association. This extra-judiciary body is the only organization charged with examining patient complaints. Out of a total of 2320 medical errors, 661 complaints were upheld, 1581 were judged unfounded and 78 were without conclusion. Half of these reports dealt with surgery.[46]

A study from the University of Basle showed a 15 per cent error rate in the administration of medicines in hospitals.[47] Hospital admissions due to adverse drug reactions have been studied prospectively in two hospitals. In the University Hospital of Lausanne over a six-month period, 7 per cent of 3195 consecutive hospital admissions were considered drug related.[48] Similarly, 6.4 per cent of all patients hospitalized in one year in a hospital in Ticino presented with an adverse drug reaction.[49] A 1999 study in the Romandie revealed that among patients attending the University Hospital of Lausanne, only 57 per cent had received a clear explanation of how to use unfamiliar medication.[12]

Participation in policy making

The direct democratic system in Switzerland allows citizens individually or in association to propose modifications of the law or constitution. There have been several plebiscites aimed at modifying the law on sickness insurance. In late 2000, a plan to limit the statutory sickness insurance to hospital costs was rejected by 82 per cent of the voters. Other initiatives are still pending, for instance using value-added tax (VAT) to pay for health care expenses or calculating insurance premiums on the basis of actual income. This last proposal seems to be supported by a large proportion of the population.[6]

Although 80 per cent of hospital directors and 94 per cent of cantonal health department heads approve of some form of rationing in health care, the general population (53 per cent) is less supportive of measures that would reduce current services.[21] Many experts argue that the Swiss have been 'spoiled' by a very comprehensive sickness insurance that keeps expectations high.

In reality, however, people remain very sensitive to rising costs in insurance premiums, and many are open to cost savings in health care. However, heated discussions about expensive medication, such as recombinant coagulation factor VIII, showed that from the consumer perspective cost plays a minor role when it comes to a question of life or death. In recent years, the rationing debate has become very important. It is universally agreed that the debate must take place openly and publicly, and any decisions should arise, according to Swiss tradition, from societal consensus.

A study of attitudes towards rationing among senior citizens in Zurich found that the criteria that was considered most important was patients' preferences, followed by treatment effectiveness.[50] Respondents in that and another study rejected the idea of using personal characteristics, such as age or nationality, as criteria for deciding who should receive treatment.[21, 50] Experts and patients alike appear to agree that effectiveness, in terms of future quality of life, and cost-effectiveness are important criteria for prioritization. However, lay people consistently rate the wishes of the patient as most important. The debates on rationalization and rationing reveal a measure of agreement between experts and the public on reducing unnecessary diagnostic tests and/or marginally effective therapies.[51]

FOCUS GROUPS

Nine focus groups were conducted between June and August 2001, details of which are shown in Table 9.1.

Table 9.1 The focus groups in the Swiss study

Group	No. of partici-pants	Age	Sex	Location	Health status
1	3	18–30	Male	Lausanne (French)	Healthy
2	10	50–65	Female	Lausanne (French)	Chronic illness
3	10	30–50	Female	Nyon (French)	Healthy
4	10	50–65	Male	Vallorbe (French)	Healthy
5	4	18–30	Female	Aigle (French)	Healthy
6	7	18–30	Female	Zurich (German)	Healthy
7	8	50–65	Male	Zurich-Hongg (German)	Chronic illness
8	11	30–50	Female	Zurich (German)	Recent inpatient
9	5	30–50	Male	Sankt-Gallen (German)	Healthy

NOTES

1 Narring, F. and Michaud, P.A. (2000) Adolescents and ambulatory care: results from a national survey of young people 15 to 20 years of age in Switzerland, *Arch Pediatr* 7(1): 25–33.

2 Gehri, M. (1997) L'enfant et l'hôpital [dossier], *La Tribune du GHRV*, 30: 2–7.

3 Manifest für eine faire Mittelverteilung in Gesundheitswesen (1999) *Intercura*, 65: 17–36.

4 Peters, M., Müller, V. and Luthiger, P. (2001) *Auswirkungen des Krankenversicherungsgesetzes auf die Versicherten*. Bern: Bundesamt für Sozial Verischerung (BSV).

5 Domenighetti, G. (1997) *Estime des Suisses pour leur système sanitaire; comparaison avec les pays de l'UE [Union européenne]*. Sécurité Sociale (Office Fédéral de la Santé Publique), 5: 279–81.

6 L'image de la médecine suisse auprès de la population: résultats d'un sondage d'opinion réalisé par l'Institut Link sur la demande de la Société médicale de la Suisse romande (1994) *Schweiz Rundschau Medizin (Praxis)*, 83(6): 169–71.

7 Gilliand, P. (1999) Démographie médicale et vieillissement de la population en Suisse, *Cahiers de Sociologie et de Démographie Médicales*, 39(4): 289–312.

8 Rossi, I. (1999) Cultural mediation and training of healthcare professionals: from cross-culture to co-discipline, *Soz Praventivmed*, 44(6): 288–294.

9 Sessa, C. *et al.* (1996) The last 3 months of life of cancer patients: medical aspects and role of home-care services in southern Switzerland, *Support Care Cancer*, 4(3): 180–5.

10 Imboden, C., Heusser, M., Jucken, H. *et al.* (1995) Das schweizerische Gesundheitswesen im Jahr 2005, in J. Kettiger, S. Magnaguagno, B. Ryf and R. Ziegler (eds) *Schweizerische Gesellschaft für Gesundheitspolitik*. Ernst & Young Consulting.

11 Gemeinsame Kommission H+KSK (2000) *Ergebnisse der zweiten strukturierten Qualitätsberichterstattung 1999*. Bern: Nationale Koordinations- und Informstionsstelle für Qualitätsförderung H+KSK.

12 Résultats de l'enquête de satisfaction 1999: 90% des patients hospitalisés recommanderaient le CHUV à leurs proches (2000) *CHUV magazine*, 9: 6–15.

13 Perneger, T.V. *et al.* (1996) Comparison of patient satisfaction with ambulatory visits in competing healthcare delivery settings in Geneva, Switzerland, *Journal of Epidemiology and Community Health*, 50(4): 463–8.

14 Grol, R. *et al.* (2000) Patients in Europe evaluate general practice care: an international comparison, *British Journal of General Practice*, 50(11): 882–7.

15 Buchs, L. (2001) Managed care, in G. Kocher and W. Oggier (eds),

Système de santé suisse 2001/2002: survol de la situation actuelle. Concordat des assureurs-maladies suisses, pp. 124–35, Soleure.

16 Page, J., Somaini, B., Jaccard, R. and Weber, R. (2000) *Quality of life and patient satisfaction among HIV-infected individuals treated by private care physicians or by specialists at an HIV-outpatient clinic* (poster). XIII International AIDS Conference, Durban, South Africa.

17 Organization for Economic Co-operation and Development (OECD) (2000). *OECD Health Data 2000: A Comparative Analysis of 29 Countries* (CD-ROM). Paris: OECD.

18 Ordonnance du 27 juin 1995 sur l'assurance-maladie (OAMal), 832.102 (1995), http://www.admin.ch/ch/f/rs/c832_102.html.

19 Loi fédérale du 18 mars 1994 sur l'assurance-maladie (LAMal), 832.10 (1994) RO (1995) 1328 (2000), http://www.admin.ch/ch/f/rs/c832_10.html.

20 Bertrand, D. and Stalder, H. (2000) Droits de l'homme et inégalité de l'accès aux soins, *Medicine and Hygiene*, 2316: 1914–20.

21 Domenighetti, G. and Maggi, J. (2000) *Définition des priorités sanitaires et rationnement: 'opinion des Suisses, des administrateurs hospitaliers et des départements sanitaires des cantons.* Lausanne: Département D'économétrie et D'économie Politique.

22 Martin, J. (1997) Le système de santé suisse: une période de mutation, *Actualité et Dossier en Santé Publique*, 21: 13–18.

23 Sprumont, D. (2001) *Effectivité des normes applicables dans la relation patient-médecin*, personal communication.

24 Brink-Muinen, A. *et al.* (2000) Doctor-patient communication in different European healthcare systems: relevance and performance from the patients' perspective, *Patient Educ Couns*, 39(1): 115–27.

25 Sanchez-Menegay, C. and Stalder, H. (1994) Do physicians take into account patients' expectations? *Journal of General Internal Medicine*, 9(7): 404–6

26 Friedemann, M.L. (1997) Do nurse clinicians influence the working climate and the quality of care? 2 results, *Pflege*, 10(3): 132–7.

27 Faisst, K., Schilling, J. and Gutzwiller, F. (2000) Quality of dispensation of prescription medication from the patients' point of view, *Schweizerische Medizinische Wochenschrift*, 130(12): 426–34

28 Demartines, N. *et al.* (2000) Telemedicine: perspectives and multi-disciplinary approach, *Schweizerische Medizinische Wochenschrift*, 130(9): 314–23.

29 Deluze, C. and Vischer, T.L. (1996) Interactions entre médecine académique et médecines non conventionnelles: étude et réflexions sur l'acupuncture, *Cahiers Médico-sociaux*, 40: 33–40.

30 Messerli-Rohrbach, V. (2000) Personal values and medical preferences: post-materialism, spirituality, and the use of complementary medicine, *Forsch Komplementarmed Klass Naturheilkd*, 7(4): 183–9.

31 Ammann, Y. (2000) *Rapport sur les principaux résultats du sondage: santé et information (sanimedia).* Service cantonal de recherche et

d'information statistiques du Canton de Vaud (SCRIS). Lausanne: SCRIS.

32 Meier, V. and Grau, P. (2001) *Alternativmedizin: Theoretische Ueberlegungen.* Bern: Krankenkasse KBB.

33 SIAK Network for Cancer Predisposition Testing and Counselling (2001). Bern: SIAK, http://www.siak.ch/_engl/services/siak/network_genetic/intro.htm.

34 Hochreutener, M.K. and Eichler, K. (2000) *Schlussbericht Outcome 98.* Zurich: Verein Outcome.

35 Diezi, J. (2001) Automedication: un besoin d'information et de formation, in T. Buclin and C. Ammon (eds), *L'automédication: Pratique Banale, Motifs Complexes. Cahiers Médico-sociaux.* Genève: Médecine et Hygiène.

36 Stuckelberger, A. (2001) Polymédication et automédication chez la personne âgée: résultats du programme national de recherche 'Vieillesse', in T. Buclin and C. Ammon (eds), *L'automédication: Pratique Banale, Motifs Complexes. Cahiers Médico-sociaux,* pp. 47–67. Genève: Médecine et Hygiène.

37 *I Tuoi Diritti Come Paziente* (1990) Bellinzona: Dipartimento delle Opere Sociali e l'Ordine dei Medici, del Cantone Ticino.

38 Messerli-Rohrbach, V. and Schaer, A. (1999) Complementary and conventional medicine: prejudices against and demands placed on natural care and conventional doctors, *Schweizerische Medizinische Wochenschrift,* 129(42): 1535–44.

39 Sanchez-Menegay, C. and Stalder, H. (1994) Do physicians take into account patients' expectations? *Journal of General Internal Medicine,* 9(7): 404–6.

40 Domenighetti, G. *et al.* (1993) Revisiting the most informed consumer of surgical services: the physician-patient, *International Journal of Technology Assessment in Healthcare,* 9(4): 505–13.

41 Sprumont, D. (1998) Droit des patients: survol de la législation, *Plädoyer,* 4: 41–6.

42 Riesen, A., Himmelberger, R., Saurer, A. and Sauvin, B. (1997) *Droits des Patients,* 2nd edn. Genève: Forum Santé.

43 Werro, F. (1996) *La Responsabilité Civile Médicale: Vers une Dérive à L'américaine?* Neuchâtel: Institut de Droit de la Santé.

44 Brunner, H.H., Conen, D., Günter, P. *et al.* (2001) Towards a safe healthcare system: Proposal for a national programme on patient safety improvement for Switzerland, http://www.swiss-q.org/apr-2001/docs/Final_ReportE.pdf.

45 La Fondation Organisation Suisse des Patients et Assurés (OSP) (2000) *Rapport d'activité 2000 23.* Zurich: OSP.

46 Kuhn, H.P. (2000) Bureau d'expertises de la FMH: rapport annuel 1999, *Bulletin des Médecins Suisses,* 81(36): 2003–6.

47 *Tribune Patienten Zeitung* (2001) La qualité: étudier les erreurs de traitement, 1: 9.

48 Livio, F., Buclin, T., Yersin, B. *et al.* (1998) *Hospitalisations Pour Effet Indésirable Médicamenteux: Recensement Prospectif Dans un Service D'urgences Médicales.* Lausanne: Institut Universitaire de Médecine Sociale et Préventive (raisons de santé 23).

49 Lepori, V., Perren, A. and Marone, C. (1999) Adverse internal medicine drug effects at hospital admission, *Schweizerische Medizinische Wochenschrift*, 129(24): 915–22.

50 Shelling, H.R. and Wettstein, A. (2000) Einstellungen von Seniorinnen und Senioren zur Rationierung im Gesundheitswesen-vor und nach einer Vorlesungsreihe, *Praxis* 89: 1200–10.

51 Werner, K. (2000) Sichtweisen und Lösungsansätze zur Kosteneindämmung im Schweizerischen Gesundheitswesen, thesis. Universities of Basel, Bern and Zurich.

10

UNITED KINGDOM[1]

OPINIONS ABOUT THE HEALTH CARE SYSTEM

The present system

The NHS continues to be at the centre of political debate in the UK and the government has recently made commitments to major increases in funding. The current health policy agenda includes quicker, more flexible access to treatment, an increased emphasis on primary care, the further integration of health and social care, greater patient involvement and new roles for health professionals. The National Institute for Clinical Excellence (NICE) and national service frameworks now set health service standards. These are delivered by clinical governance, underpinned by professional self-regulation and monitored by the Commission for Health Improvement (CHI), using the new national performance assessment framework and the national surveys of NHS patients. The overall direction of health policy is towards a primary-care led health service. Responsibility for commissioning and providing services at the local level has been devolved to Primary Care Trusts (PCTs).

Access and responsiveness

There is considerable evidence that the British public is concerned about the length of time they have to wait for treatment, in particular waiting times for hospital appointments and treatment.[2] Focus group participants confirmed that by far the most frustrating experience of the NHS is that of waiting. Waiting means not being in control, getting anxious, wasting time and generally feeling unimportant: *'My child waited seven months to have a hernia operation even though the doctor said that it needed to be done as soon as possible'*.

People fear that long waiting times impact on their health. More than a third of people referred by their GP to a hospital doctor said their condition worsened while waiting for the appointment.[3]

The current government has put reducing waiting times at the top of its agenda for reforming the NHS. Many initiatives are underway to scrutinize patient pathways and increase the speed at which they are processed through the system. Attempts to increase capacity and remove the log jams have included reforming professional roles to reduce waiting times – for example, by giving nurses more responsibilities for prescribing. The private sector is also expected to play an increasing role and the government has signed an agreement with the independent sector that stresses the importance of using spare capacity in private hospitals.

Participants in the focus groups were beginning to notice changes in the way things worked at their local health centre and hospital. Some had noticed changes in the appointments system at their GP's surgery: they can get seen more quickly if they are willing to consult any GP in the practice, rather than just the one they are registered with. Changes had also occurred in hospital accident and emergency departments with the introduction of triage systems which prioritize patients according to the severity of their symptoms.

Changes that speed up the waiting process were welcomed on the whole – *'There is a priority card system now at casualty, you see a nurse as soon as you go in'* – but some participants were critical of the NHS for providing less of a personal service than it used to: *'I think the personal touch has gone now. You don't feel like you can go in and actually discuss that you might have a problem. You just get a five-minute slot with the doctor now'*.

New processes for contracting out certain areas of the service were also seen as detrimental – a way of cutting corners rather than improving the quality of the service: *'Like cleaners – they've been put onto contract cleaning and they've only got so much time to do the job'*.

Only a small proportion of the population (about 11 per cent) has private health insurance, and almost everyone uses the NHS for the majority of their health care, but the private sector is an important benchmark of comparison for the NHS.[4] First and foremost, patients see the main benefit of using private health care as speed of access. It also offers more comfortable and pleasant surroundings with 'hotel services' that frequently far exceed those available in the NHS. Time spent with staff is another important quality factor provided by the private sector. Underlying all these points is the sense that patients are treated more as customers in the private sector, whereas they too often feel they have to 'do battle' with the NHS to get what they want out of it. However, patients do not see private health care as infallible. While it may offer quicker access and a nicer environment, few patients believe the private sector provides better clinical care. Patients also perceive that the NHS often has to pick up the pieces when things go wrong in the private sector.

Participants felt that the NHS was still under great pressure, under-resourced and understaffed: *'They are running out of money aren't they? Because they are closing wards and everything, they can't afford to man them can they, and the staff aren't getting paid what they are entitled to'*.

Media coverage of medical errors and cases of malpractice has also contributed to the erosion of public confidence in the health service: *'They've got to do something about building up trust. There are so many stories in the press now about doctors found out after years of malpractice'*.

Focus group participants frequently described their own experiences of the NHS as patchy. When it worked well it could be brilliant. Importantly, a 'good' experience of the NHS was often dependent on the way the patient had been treated by health professionals. Positive reports were more likely if they felt they had been well cared for, listened to and given sufficient time: *'When my father died earlier this year his GP couldn't have been better. He came round in his own time to see how Dad was getting on and how Mum was coping'*. However, when the system doesn't work well it was described as frustrating, time-consuming, frightening, inefficient and unable to make you better: *'My son had an accident and had a really bad broken leg. He'd had two operations and there was blood all over the sheets. I came in the next day and he was still lying on those sheets on the bed'*.

In terms of what participants themselves wanted to see in the future, many offered a simple solution for getting the NHS back on track: more staff, less bureaucracy, more money, more of a customer focus and more user-friendly hours: *'The NHS has to promote and sell itself back to the public as if it's a viable business. At the moment their reputation is completely shattered. There has to be a way of marketing that company back to us. We're its customers'*.

Few were optimistic about the future of health care in the UK.

The NHS is not meeting their expectations fully at the moment and, although they recognized that changes are taking place, they were sceptical of the capacity of the service to meet their future needs.

Structure and organization

Patients want more flexible access to health care, including access to services outside traditional working hours. Public demand for out-of-hours services was recently explored through the government's People's Panel (a representative sample of 5000 members of the public aged 16 and over).[5] Some 28 per cent of panel members said they wanted NHS hospitals to be open 24 hours a day, seven days a week for services other than emergencies. A third said they wanted GP surgeries to have extended opening hours during the week. The main reason why people want after hours access to public services is that they do not like managing their personal business at work.

Many focus group participants were attracted to the idea of a more flexible appointments system that would allow access to different doctors in order to be seen more quickly. This might involve patients being able to access any one of a group of doctors either at their local surgery or within their area, rather than being tied to a particular doctor: '*If you've got somewhere where you can go where you would see a bank of people in a more open format and get advice quicker, then fine, yes that's got to be right*'.

Some walk-in health centres have been established in England, but the concept received a fairly negative response from some focus group participants, suggesting that while patients may not want to be tied to seeing the same doctor every time, they value the familiarity of their local surgery or health centre. Some people associated walk-in centres with services for homeless people or drug users and on this basis assumed that they would be run-down and of poor quality. Patients would require reassurance about the experience and qualifications of the health professionals working in such walk-in centres: '*You get all sorts of practices on the side of the street and you pay to go in and see them. They haven't got your records have they? Not only that, they are also saying that most of them haven't done the qualifications that they have got written up on the wall*'.

There was a level of trust in the traditional model of the health professional acting as gatekeeper to the next level of more specialist expertise, although more immediate access to health professionals 'off-the-street' did appeal to some patients, particularly men: *'If you've got a back problem, for example, then what's the point in going to see your GP? He's not going to make you better. You could cut out some of the filtering system by going to the specialist straight away'.*

Cost and efficiency

The likelihood that the NHS would continue to offer universal access to comprehensive treatment and care, largely free at the point of use, was viewed pessimistically. While there was strong support for these fundamental principles, people felt that UK patients would probably have to pay more to receive services in the future. Rising prescription charges and the introduction of charges for dental services were taken as indications of 'the way things are going'. Many were also conscious of rationing of medicines and other treatments. People felt that treatment decisions were sometimes influenced by budgetary considerations as much as by consideration of clinical effectiveness.

For many the expectation of having to pay more in the future was married to a belief that there is currently a push towards encouraging more patients to take out private health insurance. There was little support for a privatized system, but some participants feared it might become inevitable: *'I think after a while you lose interest in the NHS and you tend to think about going private'.* Despite this, few people appeared to be seriously planning ahead for this eventuality; those with private insurance cover were very much in the minority. A number of participants mentioned the exclusions that accompany private health insurance – for example, the difficulty of getting treatment for a pre-existing condition.

Equity

In spite of their pessimism about the prospects for the comprehensiveness and adequacy of care, there was strong support for NHS values of universal, equitable access to health care based on need rather than the ability to pay: *'I think it's got to go more private hasn't it . . . But I don't think politically you should go down that road too far . . . there's a lot of pride in the National Health'.*

Despite their concerns, most participants expected the NHS to be there for them in some form in the future.

PATIENTS' VIEWS OF HEALTH PROFESSIONALS

Doctors

The quality of the doctor-patient relationship is central to patient's perceptions of the care they receive. Greater patient satisfaction has been associated with more use of patient-centred communications (giving information and counselling) and less doctor-centred communication (giving directions and asking questions).[6] However, a major barrier to achieving patient-centred care in the UK is the lack of time available – the average consultation time in general practice is currently less than ten minutes.

A national survey of general practice patients revealed that younger people, especially younger women, were more likely to say that GPs do not provide them with enough information.[2] Younger people were less likely to think GPs spent enough time with them and women under 25 tended to be the most critical. People from minority ethnic groups were more doubtful about their GP making the right diagnosis and consequently more likely to want a second opinion. The worse a person's self-reported health status, the more critical they were of their GP's willingness or ability to answer questions.

GPs have traditionally been the foundation of the UK's system of health care, playing a key role in ensuring continuity of care. But a national survey of general practice patients found that only 47 per cent thought their GP knew *'a lot'* about their medical history, while 37 per cent thought they knew *'a fair amount'*. There was evidence among the focus group participants that the doctor-patient tie is less sacrosanct than it is often held to be, particularly among younger age groups. Most patients, particularly men and those in the younger age groups, said that in the majority of situations they would be happy to consult anyone as long as they 'know what they are doing'. This was particularly true for minor conditions, repeat prescriptions and recurring symptoms. Furthermore, people recognized that access to different doctors meant exposure to different ways of doing things: *'My personal opinion is that it doesn't matter which GP I have . . . but I know that my mum would prefer the GP she's been with for the longest rather than the newer one that's just joined the surgery.'*

Continuity *was* desired in the treatment of ongoing, more serious conditions where participants often wanted the reassurance of speaking to someone who understood their condition and knew their history of dealing with it. They also still wanted to be able to choose to see their 'own' doctor but recognized that this could mean a longer wait for an appointment: *'It depends if you've got a history doesn't it? If you're really ill or have been really ill and the doctor knows you really well then you would prefer to see him wouldn't you?'*

Nurses

Breaking down the barriers between the responsibilities of different health professionals is part of a drive to enable the NHS to work more flexibly in the UK. The majority of focus group participants were happy with the notion of increasing the responsibility of both nurses and pharmacists as long as they received more training.

The willingness to consult different health professionals for advice and treatment was linked to a desire to be 'given time'. Time is a rare commodity in the NHS: many described having only a five-minute slot with their doctor or feeling that a hospital visit was equivalent to being on a conveyor belt. It was felt that a nurse or a pharmacist was likely to have more time to spend with them and they often felt more comfortable talking to nurses in particular: *'You'd feel like they've got time to discuss a problem. Whereas the GP you feel is always under pressure to get through the patients'*.

Nurses have taken on increased responsibilities over recent years in the UK and this trend is set to continue. Focus group participants viewed nurses as hard working and caring and it was felt that they build up experience that equips them to take more of a decision making role on prescriptions. Many patients had already noticed nurses taking on more responsibility in local health centres and were comfortable with this development: *'The experienced nurse at our surgery has already worked with the GP for the last ten years. She's very helpful'*.

Participants could also see the logic of relying on nurses to take on a broader range of responsibilities. It frees up doctors' time and access to nurses is likely to be quicker than access to doctors: *'You'd probably have greater access because it must be cheaper to run a nurse than a doctor so you'd have more nurses'*.

Some felt nurses should be allowed to prescribe a greater range of treatments: *'It's a shame they can't prescribe because I think some of them are so well qualified that they know exactly what's wrong because they see people all the time'*. However, they did not want to see nurses overburdened or poorly rewarded as a result of taking on more work. Other participants mentioned the importance of nurses having the qualifications and experience to take on more responsibility; some preferred to maintain the need for a doctor's signature on prescriptions. It was also considered important that the nurse did not become a barrier between the patient and the doctor: *'You wouldn't want the nurse to turn around and say "No I am afraid you are not seeing the doctor". If you really want to see the doctor then you book an appointment to see him'.*

Pharmacists

The majority of focus group participants had approached their pharmacist for advice and information about symptoms and treatments. Some placed considerable reliance on this advice: *'My in-laws are in their seventies and they totally rely on their pharmacist, they very rarely go to their doctors. They are at one of these surgeries where you have to wait about a week to get an appointment'.*

Pharmacists were considered experts, not shopkeepers, by many participants. They are held in high esteem and their expertise is valued, particularly in relation to minor ailments and conditions. Some people were already noticing changes at their local pharmacist, including computer records of previous prescriptions: *'I think Lloyds chemists do you a printout of what medicines you've had in the past. If all the chemists used that system you'd be able to say look, I've had this before, can I have it again?'*

There are also more negative reasons for consulting the pharmacist: because they cannot get an appointment with their GP or because they are afraid of being ridiculed or fobbed off by the doctor.[7]

Opinions differed over whether pharmacists should be allowed to prescribe. Some participants said they would be happy for them to prescribe medicines within proper guidelines, but others felt that responsibility should only extend to repeat prescriptions. Some people were concerned that pharmacists would be unwilling to take on the responsibility and liability for prescribing a broader range of medicines.

ALTERNATIVE WAYS OF ACCESSING HEALTH ADVICE

Telephone

The government has recently established a telephone helpline, NHS Direct, accessible 24 hours a day and staffed by nurses. Responses to the existing NHS Direct phone line were extremely positive among those who had used the service – in particular parents on behalf of their children:

> *My little boy had a terrible temperature ... it was six in the morning or something and I phoned up to see whether I should take him into the hospital and she took all his symptoms and everything, told me what to do to cool him down. She said 'I will ring you back in two hours to see how he is' ... and on the dot, two hours later she rang back.*

The service is becoming quite popular, but a number of focus group participants were wary of greater use of the telephone for medical consultations. While the telephone was seen to have its place for repeat prescriptions and straightforward advice and information, many were nervous of using it for more complex consultations. They felt they would be unable to describe their symptoms effectively over the phone and worried that without face-to-face contact the doctor might miss something or misinterpret their symptoms. The anonymity of a telephone consultation was also seen as a drawback; patients would want reassurance that they were speaking to a professional and not a 'bogus' doctor: *'No, it's totally wrong. I don't think people can explain properly and the doctor can't check. The doctor can easily give the wrong medicine'.*

There was also a desire for recourse if bad advice is given: *'Do they record your call? The patient should know that if something goes wrong with the advice or information they've been given they can trace the call back to the individual who gave them the advice'.* On the other hand, participants were also quick to recognize that using the telephone might be a way of accessing advice and information more quickly and reducing the burden on hospitals and health centres: *'I've got the number [NHS Direct] by the phone. I'd rather call them than get the doctor out'.*

However, many people were not aware of NHS Direct, particularly men, ethnic minorities and those in the younger age groups, and felt it should be advertised and promoted more widely. Some of the younger men were wary of using the telephone and felt they would be more likely to go straight to casualty in an emergency.

Telemedicine

At present telemedicine is only used experimentally in the UK, but research suggests it has considerable potential in certain situations.

A review of studies of patient satisfaction with teleconsultations using real time interactive videos found that patients saw distinct advantages because telemedicine offers faster access to specialist advice.[8] But telemedicine received a lukewarm response from focus group participants, largely because few could imagine how it might work in practice. Those who had seen demonstrations of tele-medicine were more positive, suggesting that it is unfamiliarity and lack of knowledge rather than opposition to telemedicine per se that makes patients sceptical of its impact: *'If it's saving time and money then yeah, it's a good thing'*; *'I went to one specialist and he sort of photographed whatever and sent it off round the world to get other views on it'*.

Those who were more sceptical were concerned about the accuracy of an assessment made without first-hand examination. Older participants in particular tended to stress the importance and value of physical examinations as the lynchpin of medical diagnoses. Furthermore, telemedicine was seen to have a limited role, as only a certain range of conditions (e.g. skin conditions) would be easy to diagnose visually. One younger participant feared that the images could be abused and too easily accessed by others around the world: *'It could get abused, seriously abused. You may have a rash on your bottom or something and the next thing you know it's on the internet'*.

EXTENDING THE SCOPE OF MEDICAL CARE

Complementary therapies

A significant proportion of people in the UK currently use comple-mentary medicine and it is predicted that this proportion will increase in the future.[9] It has been suggested that every week, around 40 per cent of GPs recommend or endorse the use of complementary medicines and one in five refers their patients to these services. People use these therapies because they are seen as more patient-centred and holistic but also because more orthodox treatment may be seen as ineffective and having adverse side-effects. Paterson and Britten found that most people use complementary therapies because they want to establish a degree of control over their situ-ation.[10] A significant proportion of those who use complementary therapies are health professionals and around 80 per cent are female. Many people who use complementary medicine are well educated:

one study found the majority of users were educated to degree level.[11]

As the body of evidence supporting the value of some alternative medicines builds up, there is the possibility of making such treatments a more mainstream part of NHS services. Some focus group participants took the pragmatic approach – 'if it works, give it a go' – others were enthusiasts, and valued the concept of more natural, less intrusive approaches to health care: *'For years and years here you've only had traction for back problems . . . acupuncture, chiropractic and so on are only just coming in . . . there's been unnecessary suffering because they didn't want to recognize that other forms of treatment existed'.*

However, some viewed it as a 'second best' option that's only worth looking into if conventional medicine has failed. Others recalled scare stories they'd picked up in the media about bogus practitioners and alternative medicine that has done more harm than good: *'On this programme the other night, they were saying that anybody can set up and say they are doing you good when they are not doing anything . . . this woman had had a neck massage from someone who didn't know what he was doing and she was paralysed from the neck down'.*

Participants recognized that such treatments are on the margins of what the NHS does at the moment: *'There are some parts of the NHS who accept acupuncture. It's a last resource isn't it . . . they will let you do it, but they like to try other things first'.*

While some who had tried alternative therapies had done so on the advice of their doctor, others had taken a more hit and miss approach to finding a practitioner. The issue of trust was an important one but, beyond looking for qualifications from an authoritative body, participants had little notion of how else they might be reassured by the credentials of alternative practitioners. The majority welcomed more information about what alternatives were available and clearer guidelines on the best people to go to.

New medicines and biotechnologies

A recent survey looked at public attitudes towards the use of genetic information.[12] While nine out of ten people agreed that genetic developments should be used to diagnose and treat diseases in the future, one third were concerned that genetic research was tampering with nature and therefore unethical. Respondents with a high level of knowledge about genetics and parents of young children were more likely to be positive about the potential health benefits.

The wider availability of genetic tests for serious conditions received the most negative response of all the future scenarios presented to focus groups: *'If someone told you next year that you're going to die of cancer, would you want to know?'* Although a small minority (mainly women) were keen to equip themselves with as much knowledge about their health prospects and their children's health as possible, the majority felt that easy access to self-diagnosis tests was a step too far and would create a nation of neurotic hypochondriacs. Most felt they would only carry out such tests on the advice of a health professional: *'With too much information you can get people thinking they've got something when they haven't'.*

INFORMATION FOR PATIENTS

Health information needs

For most patients the first and most trusted information source is their doctor, although many also seek out supplementary information from a variety of sources. However, faith in doctors' expertise is beginning to be eroded. Younger patients see themselves as far more informed than the previous generation and younger middle-class people in particular no longer regard the medical profession as the fount of all knowledge.[13] There are exceptions to this trend: for example, some patients with severe conditions may be fearful of seeking out additional sources of information.[14]

While most focus group participants welcomed more information, they were a long way from feeling expert about the NHS and health care generally. The type of information they wanted included details about service quality and information about diseases and treatment options, including waiting times, success rates for particular operations and the qualifications of individual specialists. They also wanted to know who was going to perform their operation, what a treatment or operation would entail, how long it would take to recover, how long they would have to spend in hospital, what sort of medication they might need and possible side-effects. People felt generally ill informed on all these issues: *'You'd want to know as much as you could but you'd want to have that information given to you. You wouldn't want to have to go and find out for yourself . . . spending the day in the library to find out what's wrong with you'.*

Information sources

Information-gathering by participants included reading leaflets, talking to friends and family and so on. They relied heavily on information from health professionals and patient groups, but more populist sources such as magazines, newspapers, television and radio programmes were also used, particularly by women.

Some participants were more proactive in seeking out health information than others: those with chronic illnesses; parents with children at home (the only people in the focus groups who had used NHS Direct); women; and, to a lesser extent, older age groups and those with hospital experience: *'It seems to me that GPs, they can't read every bit of information and they've got to make all these decisions so why shouldn't we get involved?'*

Men in the focus groups were consistently less proactive when describing their approach to finding out about health. The reasons for this differed between the age groups. The younger men felt that, beyond having a very vague awareness of the importance of healthy eating and fitness, it wasn't relevant to them. The older age groups, particularly those in the 50–65 category, were heavily reliant on others telling them what to do. There was an underlying feeling that health issues were, to an extent, 'women's issues': *'I'm not really that active about finding out about health stuff, it's usually when something happens and I just go and look into it. It's not an issue until it goes wrong'.*

Younger people (18–30s) tended to be less active in seeking information about health issues, unless they had a chronic illness, had developed a particular condition or had children. Youth itself was seen as a reason not to be too bothered about health issues and many were quite complacent about the need to be informed: *'Except for recently with the acne thing, I don't really see any reason to go and look for information'.*

At the same time, however, younger people were more likely to question the advice they were given by health professionals and were less tied to the 'doctor knows best' model of thinking. They might be prompted into action if they picked up on an issue in the media or if they felt they were getting a poor response from their doctor. Younger participants also felt more confident about how to find information for themselves and were most at ease about using new technology to do this: *'I've been very docile about checking up on the things that I've been taking until recently, with all the scandals that have been going on you know'.*

Attitudes towards finding out about medicines were mixed and sometimes contradictory. On the one hand, many participants claimed to be vigilant about reading drug information leaflets. Many spoke to their pharmacist before buying over-the-counter medicines and also asked them about prescribed medicines, as they tended not to get this information from their doctor: '*I think you get more information about the tablets you are being given from the pharmacy than you do the doctor*'.

On the other hand, there was a perception that it was impossible to know everything and that a level of trust needs to be placed in the health professional who has prescribed the medication: '*You just tend to take it, you trust the doctors judgement and take it . . . if it's got a side-effect you'll soon find out*'.

Health websites

Less than a handful of participants in the focus groups had consulted the internet for information about health issues. Some, particularly in the younger age groups, could see the benefit of being able to access a broad and diverse range of information and the potential to find out about new ideas and practices: '*Well a lot of these you can access and they print documents in relation to a condition. You can print them off, you've got access to it direct. I found it brilliant*'.

Few participants said they would welcome online consultations. Furthermore, the internet was seen as a supplement to, rather than a replacement for, more traditional paper-based information sources. People from ethnic minority groups are less likely to have access to the internet at home, as are older people and those in lower socioeconomic groups, but access via the television may help to bridge this gap.

There was some concern about the reliability of health information on the internet, although this could be overcome by looking for 'official', national websites such as NHS Direct Online, or recognized patient group sites: '*Maybe the NHS could set up its own internet site. You would tend to trust that more than you would anything else*'.

In the future it is possible that patients may access more advice and information from health professionals via email. The response of focus group participants to this development was largely negative. Some were concerned that they wouldn't be able to decipher a written response as it would involve medical terms. Email was considered to be more anonymous than using the telephone and the credentials of the sender would be uncertain. Email also offered less of an immediate response and a slow email system might exacerbate this:

> *You can speak faster than you can write can't you? I would rather speak to someone . . . you can gauge the sort of person you are talking to by the way they talk back to you.*

> *I'm not very good at all at writing letters to begin with so . . . and you just don't trust the person you are writing to is actually answering your emails and not his mum or somebody!*

One participant was also concerned that using email could be open to abuse: *'I'd be worried about who they'd give that information to . . . would it go to the drug companies? It's not very secure'*. However, there were a few positive comments. Patients could use email if they desired anonymity, it might be a way of finding out information following a consultation, and some could imagine using email for a second opinion: *'It could keep it quite anonymous couldn't it? There may be some things you wouldn't want to ask face-to-face'*.

PATIENT EMPOWERMENT

Self-diagnosis, self-medication, self-care

One UK study of over 500 patients found that around half of the illness episodes recorded by patients during a four-week period resulted in self-care alone, 17 per cent resulted in self- and professional care and 5 per cent in professional care alone.[15] The notion of self-care received a mixed response from focus groups. Participants recognized that they had responsibility for certain areas of their own care, particularly eating healthily and keeping fit, but more advanced models of self-care (e.g. self-monitoring of blood pressure or cholesterol) were was seen as a more alien and difficult concepts.

Most participants felt relatively knowledgeable about when they could look after themselves without having to see a doctor. They tended to wait a few days, trying a method of treating themselves, speaking to their pharmacist and so on before making a doctor's appointment: *'I do believe that we will sit and nurse ourselves for two or three days prior to going to the doctor'*; *'I think most people don't go unless they have to do they? Unless it's children. I think with a child you'd rather take them to see a doctor'*.

Men in particular seemed more likely to ride out an illness and hold back from seeing their doctor, others also feared being made to feel as if they had wasted the doctor's time with a minor complaint. The vast majority of participants in the focus groups felt relatively knowledgeable about healthy eating and healthy living issues. Many described the steps they took individually and on behalf of their families: taking vitamin supplements, trying to eat well and doing some exercise: *'The doctor told me I need to exercise – that's what helps the heart pump the blood around and carries all the impurities out. So I thought, if that's what I've got to do then that's what I'll do . . . I took up exercise and I've never felt better'.* However, for the majority these measures were adopted in a half-hearted manner: *'We eat sensibly but we're also only human and we do stray occasionally you know . . . occasionally you can't go past a burger bar or kebab shop, you know for lunch'.*

Even those patients living with chronic illnesses described scenarios where they were heavily dependent on their doctors or specialist to keep them on track: *'It's your responsibility to eat the right foods, exercise, stay healthy. It's the doctor's responsibility to make sure you do it'.*

There were signs however that some participants were carrying out self-care responsibilities beyond coping with minor illnesses and trying to lead a healthy lifestyle. Some of the younger men talked of checking their blood pressure and fitness levels at the gym on a regular basis. Others were conscious of family illnesses and were vigilant in checking for the symptoms in themselves or their children: *'Well in my case I will go to the doctor and say I want a cholesterol test. My dad died of a massive heart attack at 42 and his brother died and his other brother died and his mother died'.*

A number of the younger male participants talked of making access to 'everyday' tests like blood pressure and cholesterol much easier – for example, by making them more available in public places like leisure centres and shops. They also felt that education was an important priority. Some in other groups felt that making a medical health check a more regular occurrence – perhaps in the same way that you go for a regular check-up at the dentist – would be beneficial in encouraging a more preventative approach to ill-health.

Involvement in treatment decisions

Very few participants in the focus groups felt in control when they came into contact with the NHS. Those who felt more confident tended to be those with more experience (i.e. those with chronic conditions or recent experience as acute patients). More commonly participants felt they were a burden on the NHS and were conscious of the limited time they could be afforded within it. Those who challenged what they had been told or the level of service they received frequently felt as if they had been labelled a 'difficult patient': *'You get the impression they're just switching off and they've already thought what to give you before you open your mouth'.*

The NHS was not felt to be patient-focused or to view people as 'customers' receiving a service. Experiences within the NHS were often described as confrontations and participants described numerous barriers they came up against along the way. These ranged from a 'difficult' receptionist at their local health centre, or the complicated language used to explain symptoms and treatments, to the feeling of having to pester people in order to get the information or feedback they were waiting for. Although individual doctors and nurses were frequently described as outstanding, participants often characterized their relationship with the system as 'them' and 'us'. The sense of powerlessness that characterized many people's experience of the NHS was largely a result of lack of information and knowledge about how things work. Participants talked of doctors and specialists using an alien language. The traditional image of the all-knowing doctor and the ill-informed but grateful patient persisted: *'They don't use simple terms, they say blah blah blah, and you think what is that? It sounds really awful'.*

The NHS was compared unfavourably in this respect with the private sector. Private health care gives patients more time and places greater importance on making sure patients' needs are met: *'In private the fact that you're paying makes them make the time to listen to you. In the NHS it's like a piece-work system – if you ask them they'll answer the question but they don't have any obligation to make you feel comfortable'.*

However, not everyone felt powerless when they came into contact with the NHS – some did take charge and find ways of getting what they wanted out of the service. They tended to be more confident, more articulate and under 50: *'I actually said "look, I'm not leaving this surgery until you sort something out" and they got me in the hospital and they couldn't believe how far it had gone, you know'.* A common theme in the focus groups was that you had to pester and chase in order to get anywhere: *'You seem to have to make a real nuisance of yourself if you want to get anywhere'.*

Participants found it difficult to imagine a more choice-based model for the NHS where the patient, armed with the right information, could play a role in deciding the course and location of treatment they wish to pursue. Most do not feel sufficiently knowledgeable or informed to establish a dialogue with the doctor rather than simply accepting what they're given. There is also a degree of reluctance to accept that sometimes there isn't always a straightforward answer – i.e. 'this medicine is best because . . .' – but instead a series of choices and trade-offs between less than perfect alternatives.

Electronic patient-held records

The future may see the replacement of paper-based medical histories with smart cards that store personal health data. The majority of people in the focus groups felt this would be a positive development and quickly made the connection between having a smart card and quicker, more flexible access to different health professionals. Participants who valued their relationship with a particular health centre felt they would still continue to go there, but those who were less concerned about this felt they would be more able to pick and choose where to go for treatment: *'It wouldn't be such a big deal anyway if you have to see a different doctor every time because at least they would know your medical history'*.

Participants were quick to point out the ease of movement between health professionals both within the UK and abroad: *'My mother is 85 and quite often she says she won't come and stay with me because she's worried about being away from her own doctor. If she had something like that, she could bring it with her so my doctor could see'*.

Many believed that a medical smart card would be no different to carrying around a credit card. It could be used by pharmacists for repeat prescriptions without the need to visit a doctor. It would give patients greater control over their records. It would cut down administration and any health professional would have quick and easy access to a patient's past medical history: *'I am allergic to penicillin and, you know, if I am ever unconscious, you know, they could pick that out straight away'*.

Issues of privacy and confidentiality were a relatively low priority and something that most felt could be covered by data protection laws or by establishing password access to information. There was also an assumption that much of their personal health information was already held on computer, since they saw their doctor using a computer during consultations.

But the idea of patients being the sole carriers of their medical histories was not welcomed; the majority wanted the reassurance of someone else also taking responsibility for keeping a record of their health. This was partly a symptom of the paternalistic health care system that currently exists in the UK, but there were also fears of losing the card or forgetting it when turning up for an appointment.

Choosing where to receive care

Most patients in the UK say they want to be treated as close to where they live as possible, but they acknowledge the need for trade-offs – for example, travelling further afield to gain faster access to treatment. The extent to which people are willing to make this trade-off depends on many factors, including the severity of their condition and the convenience of travel arrangements for themselves and their relatives or friends. Many people support moves to provide more services in their local community rather than in acute hospital settings. They like the idea of spending more time after treatment at home, as long as health professionals can visit them to ensure there are no problems.[16] A recent study found that patients using specialist outreach clinics in general practice were more satisfied than those who went to the more traditional outpatient clinic.[17]

However, the creation of centres of excellence in particular areas or the opportunity to be treated more quickly further afield may require UK patients to travel more in the future. Focus group participants considered this a worthwhile price to pay: *'It would be nice to get it on your doorstep but if you can't, I'm willing to travel'*.

Some concerns were raised. Participants did not believe they should have to travel for emergency treatment. Travelling was likely to present difficulties for older or disabled patients. A few people felt that it represented too much of a step back: *'Isn't that going backwards though? In less developed countries they have to travel for two days to see a doctor'*.

A key aim of the latest NHS reforms is to enable patients to navigate the system better. Focus group participants tended to rely on word of mouth for information about quality of care, so a more robust mechanism for measuring the performance of hospitals, health centres and individual health professionals was welcomed. Parallels were drawn with school performance rankings, which many felt helped parents to make more informed choices about their children's education: *'When I was pregnant, I spoke to friends and said "what's Lewisham Hospital like?" and "What's Greenwich Hospital like? Which should I choose? Where should I go?" These things are important . . . and it would be good if you had this sort of information to go to'.*

Participants felt that some form of NHS performance ranking would enable patients to access services outside their local area. If they knew there was a shorter waiting list for treatment in another part of the country, they could make the choice about whether to travel. Many also felt that such information would weed out bad and bogus doctors: *'Maybe if hospitals knew they were being watched by the public they'd do something about "iffy" doctors or practices'.*

There were also some concerns about the development of NHS performance rankings. More performance information could create an even more pressured environment for health professionals and might demoralize staff. There was concern that being able to evaluate health professionals could create pressure and long waiting lists for those who are excellent and less work for those with poorer reputations. For some participants, knowing more about performance variations in the NHS was likely to highlight the weaknesses of the service rather than facilitate choice: *'There should be a standard across the country for all the GPs and hospitals; you shouldn't have to travel to see the best person'.*

Access to NHS performance rankings would only be relevant to patients if they could choose – knowing that your local hospital is performing poorly in relation to others without being able to go elsewhere is unlikely to make the patient feel more in control: *'I don't see what point there would be in it quite honestly, because like we've just said, we are in this area and that's where you get sent'.*

Participants were keen to stress that performance information should be collected and disseminated by a body independent of the NHS.

NEW ROLES FOR THE CITIZEN

Strengthening patients' rights

There was a perception among the focus group participants that the NHS is difficult to challenge if something goes wrong and that patients lose out because health professionals tend to close ranks and deflect scrutiny: *'They did the wrong operation on my foot. When*

I was examined, they agreed that they had done it wrong but when it came to the solicitor dealing with it they changed what they said, even though my partner was a witness'.

Despite this, awareness of patients' rights was low and ideas about what these rights might be were only loosely formed. Some participants were aware of their rights to see their medical records and others thought they might have a right to a second opinion. By and large, however, the rights agenda has not made much impact on patients in the UK and the concept of more clearly defined patients' rights is a relatively alien one.

Participants found it relatively difficult to imagine what rights it would be useful to have in the future, although a number of suggestions were made including: the right to be spoken to in your own language, the right not to be struck off a doctor's list without a reason, the right to change doctors, the right to access medical records and the right to a second opinion.

Participation in policy making

The NHS Plan set out a range of proposals to ensure patients' views are more effectively heard throughout the service, including a new patient advice and liaison service and patients' forums in every hospital and primary care trust to provide direct patient input into how local services are run. Patients who wish to make formal complaints about the service can now do so via the new Independent Complaints Advisory Service. A new national Commission for Patient and Public Involvement will coordinate and support the work of local community groups engaged in developing, shaping and evaluating services. The Commission will employ local teams who will promote and facilitate involving the public in local decisions that affect their health. In addition, locally-elected councillors will have the right to scrutinize health policy implementation and refer any concerns to the Secretary of State for Health.

These developments are very new and had not been implemented at the time the UK research was carried out, so they did not form part of the focus group discussions.

FOCUS GROUPS

Eight groups took place in November 2000, details of which are shown in Table 10.1.

Table 10.1 The focus groups in the UK study

Group	No. of partici- pants	Age	Sex	Location	Health status
1	7	18–30	Male	Rural Cheshire	– Healthy
2	7	18–30	Female	South London	Afro-Caribbean
3	7	30–50	Male	West Midlands	Asian
4	7	30–50	Female	West Midlands	– Healthy
5	7	30–50	Female	Birmingham	Inpatient in last 3 years
6	7	30–50	Male	Essex	Inpatient in last 3 years
7	7	50–65	Female	Rural Cheshire	Chronic illness
8	7	50–65	Male	Essex	Chronic illness

NOTES

1 Some results from the UK research were previously published in Kendall, L. (2001) *The Future Patient*. London: Institute of Public Policy Research.
2 Airey, C. and Erens, B. (1999) *National Survey of NHS Patients: General Practice 1998*. London: DoH.
3 Secretary of State for Health (2000) *The NHS Plan*, Cm 4818–I. London: The Stationery Office.
4 Kendall, L. (2001) The future patient, in *Health Trends Review*, proceedings of a conference at the Barbican Centre, London, October.
5 Cabinet Office (2000) *Open all Hours*? Results from the People's Panel, Issue 5. London: Cabinet Office.
6 Williams, S., Weinman, J. and Dale, J. (1998) Doctor patient communication and patient satisfaction: a review, *Family Practice*, 15: 480–92.
7 Hassell, K., Noyce, P.R., Rogers, A., Harris, J. and Wilkinson, J. (1997) A pathway to the GP: the pharmaceutical 'consultation' as the first port of call in primary healthcare, *Family Practice*, 14(6): 498–502.
8 Mair, F. and Whitten, P. (2000) Systematic review of studies of patient satisfaction with telemedicine, *British Medical Journal*, 320: 1517–20.
9 Pahl, R. (1999) Social trends: the social context of healthy living, *Policy Futures for UK Health*, 1999 Technical Series No. 6. London: Nuffield Trust.
10 Paterson, C. and Britten, N. (1999) 'Doctors can't help much': the search for an alternative, *British Journal of General Practice*, 49: (445): 626–9.
11 Vincent, C. and Furnham, A. (1996) Why do patients turn to complementary medicine? An empirical study, *British Journal of Clinical Psychology*, 35: 37–8.

12 MORI (2001) *Survey of People's Panel Attitudes to the use of Genetic Information*. London: Cabinet Office.
13 Institute for Public Policy Research (1998) *Rights and Responsibilities*, draft report of public consultation for Policy Forum on the Future of Health and Healthcare. London: IPPR.
14 Boudioni, M. and McPherson, K. (2000) Cancer patients' information needs and information seeking behaviour: in-depth interview study, *British Medical Journal*, 320: 909–13.
15 Rogers, A., Hassell, K and Nicolaas, G. (1999) *Demanding Patients? Analysing the Use of Primary Care*. Buckingham: Open University Press.
16 Lenaghan, J. (1999) *The National Health Service, Today and Tomorrow*, report of community issue groups. London: IPPR.
17 Bowling, A., Stramer, K., Dickinson, E., Windson, J. and Bond, M. (1997) Evaluation of specialists' outreach clinics in general practice in England: process and acceptability to patients, specialists and general practitioners, *Journal of Epidemiology and Community Health*, 51: 52–61

11

COMMUNICATION, INFORMATION, INVOLVEMENT AND CHOICE

TELEPHONE SURVEY

Focus groups provide valuable insights into the way people react to and interpret particular scenarios, but since the groups are small one cannot be certain that the views expressed are representative of the populations from which they are drawn. In order to gain information from representative population samples in each of the countries, we decided to carry out a survey to explore attitudes to selected topics in much larger population samples. We developed a short questionnaire to elicit information about people's perceptions of how well health professionals communicated with them, how well-informed they felt and their sense of opportunities for involvement and choice in their health care (see Appendix c). This was written in English and translated into German, Italian, Polish, Slovenian, Spanish, Swedish and French (in Switzerland both French and German versions were used).

The fieldwork, which was organized by NIPO, a Netherlands-based market research institute, using computer-assisted telephone interviewing (random-digit dialling), took place in each of the eight countries in July 2002. About 1000 interviews were carried out in each country with random samples of the adult population (aged 16 and over) (see Table 11.1).

The results for each country were weighted afterwards to ensure that they were nationally representative in terms of the age-sex distribution. For Germany, Italy, Switzerland and the UK regional weights were also applied. The survey provided an opportunity to make direct comparisons between subgroups. We wanted to compare responses between the countries and we were also interested to see if

Table 11.1 Telephone survey: respondents by sex and age group

	Germany n	Italy n	Poland n	Slovenia n	Spain n	Sweden n	Switzerland n	UK n	Total n
Men									
16–24	72	75	125	101	131	61	50	68	683
25–34	73	95	114	82	103	65	100	93	725
35–44	99	84	105	95	72	71	99	105	730
45–54	77	101	118	87	66	64	95	75	683
55–64	76	59	52	58	55	66	65	63	494
65+	83	76	11	70	73	103	55	85	556
Women									
16–24	69	61	120	82	77	45	67	63	584
25–34	58	121	111	92	83	85	97	93	740
35–44	119	89	103	95	94	78	123	96	797
45–54	79	79	101	119	86	96	103	84	747
55–64	95	101	83	75	63	100	77	62	656
65+	126	80	7	58	97	166	69	121	724
Total	1026	1021	1050	1014	1000	1000	1000	1008	8119

there were differences between younger and older people and between those in different educational status groups, as this might be indicative of future trends.

USE OF HEALTH CARE

Attitudes to health care are likely to be influenced by the frequency with which people use it. So we began by asking interviewees whether they had used any health care in the last 12 months, and when their most recent visit took place. Women were more likely than men to have received health care in the previous 12 months (67 per cent as compared to 56 per cent), and not surprisingly older people were more likely to have made a recent visit to a health care provider: 51 per cent of those aged 55 and over had visited in the past month, as compared to 35 per cent of those aged 16–34 and 39 per cent of those aged 35–54.

Figure 11.1 shows reported rates of health care utilization by country. People in Germany were much more likely to have received

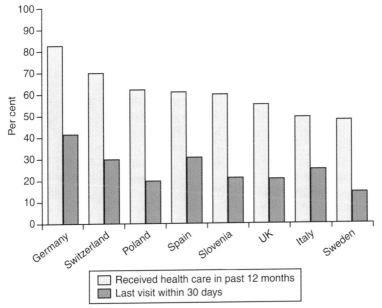

Figure 11.1   Health care utilization

health care in the previous 12 months than those in the other countries and they were also the most frequent users of health care: 81 per cent had made a visit to a health care provider in the past year, and half of these had used the service in the previous month (42 per cent of the total sample). Swedish people were at the opposite end of the spectrum, with only 50 per cent reporting a visit in the past year, only just under a third of whom had been in the past month (15 per cent of the total).

COMMUNICATIONS WITH HEALTH PROFESSIONALS

We asked people who had consulted a health professional in the previous 12 months to comment on their experience of communicating with doctors (or nurses and other health professionals if they hadn't seen a doctor). Just over half the respondents said the doctors they consulted always listened carefully to them, explained things in a way they could understand and gave them time to ask questions about their health problems or treatment. There were clear age trends in the proportion responding favourably, with a tendency for younger people to give less favourable reports than older people (see Table 11.2).

There was also a clear association between people's views on communication and their educational status: reports of doctors' communication skills were more positive from those who had received higher education than from those whose education had ceased after primary school (see Table 11.3).

The differences between the countries were striking, with respondents in Poland reporting markedly worse experience of consultations with health professionals (see Figures 11.2–11.4).

Of Polish respondents, 24 per cent said that the health providers they consulted didn't usually listen carefully to what they had to say, 31 per cent said they didn't usually provide clear explanations and 35 per cent said they didn't usually give them sufficient time to ask questions. When responses to these three questions are combined, the differences between the countries becomes even more apparent (see Figure 11.5).

Overall, 36 per cent of survey respondents said that doctors always listened carefully, gave them time to ask questions and provided full explanations. People in the UK, Switzerland, Italy and Spain gave much more favourable reports than those in Poland and Germany.

Table 11.2 Favourable reports of communication with health professionals (by age group)*

	16–24 (n = 732) %	25–34 (n = 824) %	35–44 (n = 906) %	45–54 (n = 887) %	55–64 (n = 788) %	65+ (n = 893) %	Total (n = 5030) %
Always listens carefully	50	50	51	57	58	66	55
Always allows time for questions	49	50	52	55	55	61	54
Always gives clear explanations	51	53	57	56	60	66	57

* Only includes those who had consulted a health professional within the previous 12 months

Table 11.3 Favourable reports of communication with health professionals (by educational status)*

	Primary (n = 1509) %	Secondary (n = 2465) %	University (n = 1028) %
Always listens carefully	52	57	58
Always allows time for questions	48	55	60
Always gives clear explanations	50	58	65

*   Only includes those who had consulted a health professional within the previous 12 months

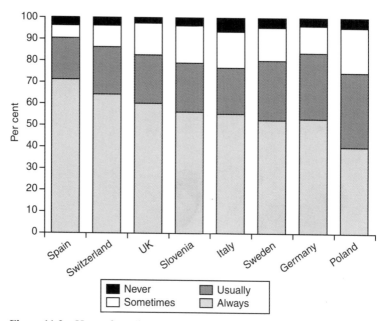

Figure 11.2   How often did doctors (or other providers) listen carefully to you?

There is sometimes a difference between what people say when they are asked to report on what happened ('experience' questions) and their opinions when they are asked to provide ratings ('satisfaction' questions). Satisfaction ratings tend to be more influenced

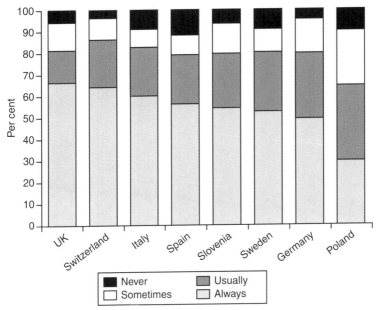

Figure 11.3 How often did doctors (or other providers) give you time to ask questions about your health problem or treatment?

by prior expectations than factual reports of specific experiences. Our survey included both types of question: questions about how often doctors listened, allowed time for questions and gave full explanations are examples of 'experience' questions, but we also asked respondents to rate how well providers communicated with them (see Figure 11.6). The 'rating' questions produced slightly different results from the 'experience' questions. This time, Switzerland achieved the highest satisfaction score but Poland again came out worst. Only 52 per cent of respondents from Poland rated communication as 'good' or 'very good', compared to 87 per cent in Switzerland, 83 per cent in Sweden and 81 per cent in the UK.

INFORMATION SOURCES

We asked respondents where, or from whom, they would normally expect to obtain information about new treatments (see Figure 11.7). Doctors were mentioned as a primary source of information by

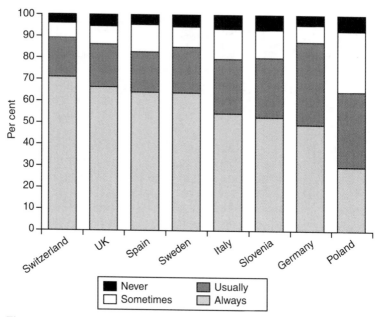

Figure 11.4   How often did doctors (or other providers) explain things in a way you could understand?

84 per cent of all respondents, with GPs mentioned by 62 per cent and specialists by 22 per cent. After doctors, newspapers and magazines were the next most popular source of information, with the internet attracting a mention from only 10 per cent of respondents. Interestingly, very few people saw patients' organizations as a source of information about new treatments.

There were considerable differences between the countries in the likelihood of mentioning the mass media as a source of information (Figure 11.8). For example, TV or radio was mentioned by 35 per cent of respondents from Slovenia, but only 2 per cent of those in Spain. People in northern European countries were much more likely to mention newspapers or magazines as a source than people in Italy or Spain. Indeed, respondents in these countries were less likely to mention any mass media source than those elsewhere.

Internet coverage is growing fast, but use of the internet to find health information is still quite uneven between our study countries. For example, it was cited as a source of information about new medicines by more than 15 per cent of respondents in Sweden,

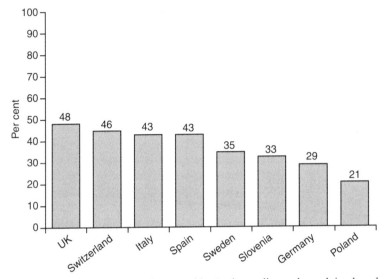

Figure 11.5   Doctors (or other providers) always listened, explained and allowed time for questions

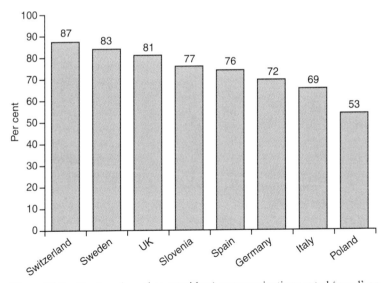

Figure 11.6   Doctors (or other providers) communications rated 'good' or 'very good'

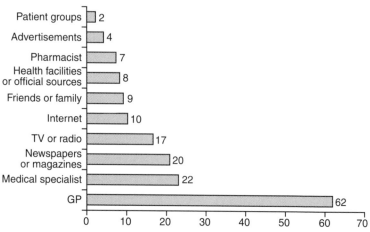

Figure 11.7   Where would you normally expect to find information about new treatments?

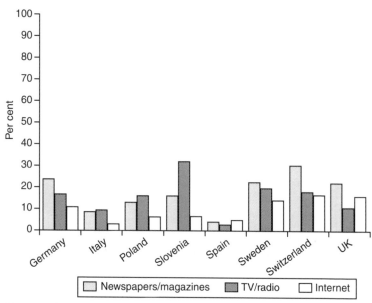

Figure 11.8   Use of mass media to find out about new treatments

Switzerland and the UK, but by only 6 per cent in Poland, Slovenia and Spain and by only 2 per cent of respondents in Italy. Not surprisingly, the internet was more frequently cited as an information source by younger people (mentioned by 14 per cent of those aged under 34, but by only 4 per cent of those aged 55 or older) and by those with more education (mentioned by 19 per cent of those educated to degree level, but by only 5 per cent of those with only primary education).

Overall, 43 per cent of respondents felt they had sufficient information about new treatments to choose the best one, while 45 per cent felt they lacked this information (see Table 11.4). Younger people were less likely to say they had sufficient information about new treatments than older people. People who had secondary or university education were somewhat more likely to respond positively (45 per cent) than those who had only primary education (40 per cent). Respondents in Switzerland were more than twice as likely as people in Poland to feel confident that they had sufficient information (see Figure 11.9).

People were asked to describe the problems they face when seeking health information. The most frequently mentioned problems

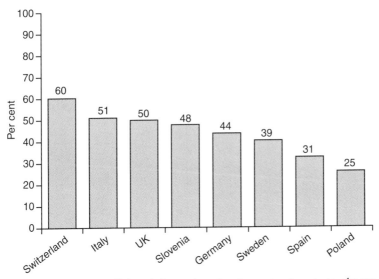

Figure 11.9   Have sufficient information about new treatments to choose the best one for me

Table 11.4 Do you feel you have sufficient information about new treatments to choose the best one for you? (by age group)

	16–24 (n = 1267) %	25–34 (n = 1465) %	35–44 (n = 1527) %	45–54 (n = 1430) %	55–64 (n = 1150) %	65+ (n = 1280) %	Total (n = 8119) %
Yes	40	37	39	43	49	55	44
No	51	52	49	45	40	31	45
Don't know/not applicable	9	11	12	12	11	14	11

Table 11.5 What do you find dissatisfying about the information available to you?*

	Total (n = 2690) %
Available information is hard to understand	40
Haven't been able to find any information	36
Available information is conflicting	14
Don't trust the information available	11
Information is insufficient, too basic, not detailed enough	8
It's not easy to find – you have to go looking for it	3
Lack of time prevents doctors supplying adequate information	3
Doctors won't/can't supply adequate information	2
Technological developments make it hard for doctors/patients to stay up to date	1

* Only includes those who mentioned a problem with information

are listed in Table 11.5. One third of respondents mentioned a problem with finding information about new treatments. Of these, just over a third said they hadn't managed to find any information relevant to their needs, while the others gave various reasons why the information available was unsatisfactory. A significant proportion of respondents said they found the available information hard to understand, while others had managed to find only conflicting or untrustworthy information.

INVOLVEMENT IN TREATMENT DECISIONS

The interviewers in each of the countries asked people for their views on who should take the lead in making treatment choices when more than one option was available. Respondents were asked to select one of five responses: the patient alone, the patient after consultation with the doctor, the doctor and patient together, the doctor after discussion with the patient or the doctor alone. These options are based on the Control Preferences Scale, developed by Degner and her colleagues, which has been used in a number of studies to determine the extent to which patients wish to be involved in decisions about their care.[1] Overall, 23 per cent saw themselves (the patient) and 26 per cent saw the doctor as the primary decision

Table 11.6 Who do you think should make the decision about which treatment is best for you? (by age group)

	16–24 (n = 1267) %	25–34 (n = 1465) %	35–44 (n = 1527) %	45–54 (n = 1430) %	55–64 (n = 1150) %	65+ (n = 1280) %	Total (n = 8119) %
I should decide	6	5	6	6	4	4	5
I should make the decision after consulting my doctor	22	22	19	17	14	12	18
My doctor and I should decide together	45	51	53	52	53	52	51
My doctor should make the decision after discussion with me	18	15	15	15	18	16	16
My doctor should decide	10	7	8	10	11	16	10

maker, but the shared decision making model, in which doctor and patient are held to be jointly responsible for making treatment decisions was the most popular, with 51 per cent of the total sample opting for it (see Table 11.6). Older people were more likely to view the doctor as the primary decision maker: 31 per cent of those aged 55 and over said the doctor should decide, compared to 24 per cent of those aged under 35.

People with higher educational status were more likely to say patients should have an active role in decision making (25 per cent) than those with secondary education (23 per cent) and those with primary education (21 per cent) (see Table 11.7). There were also notable variations between the countries (see Figure 11.10). While 91 per cent of Swiss respondents and 87 per cent of those in Germany felt the patient should have a role in treatment decisions, either sharing responsibility for decision making with the doctor or being the primary decision maker, the proportion of Polish patients who felt the same way was only 59 per cent and in Spain it was only 44 per cent. In these two countries a much higher proportion of patients felt the doctor rather than the patient should be the primary decision maker.

However, even in Poland and Spain the preference among patients for a passive role was by no means universal. More respondents in Poland (45 per cent) and Spain (38 per cent) complained that doctors failed to involve them sufficiently in decisions about their care than in any of the other countries (see Figure 11.11).

Table 11.7 Who do you think should make the decision about which treatment is best for you? (by educational status)

	Primary (n = 2464) %	*Secondary (n = 3963)* %	*University (n = 1631)* %
I should decide	5	5	7
I should make the decision after consulting my doctor	16	18	18
My doctor and I should decide together	46	52	55
My doctor should make the decision after discussion with me	19	16	14
My doctor should decide	15	9	7

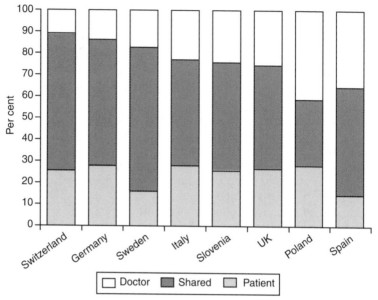

Figure 11.10   Who should have the primary role in decision making?

CHOICE OF PROVIDER

In addition to investigating the extent of desire for a role in treatment choices, we wanted to learn how far people felt they should be able to choose between different providers. The overwhelming majority of respondents felt patients ought to have a free choice of primary care doctor, specialist doctor or hospital (see Table 11.8).

Interestingly, people with higher education were slightly less likely to feel they should be able to choose specialists or hospitals than those with only primary education (see Table 11.9)

There was strong support for the notion of free choice of provider in nearly all the study countries (see Table 11.10). The one notable exception was Sweden where the majority wanted a free choice of GP, but only 31 per cent felt they should have a free choice of specialist doctor and only 54 per cent wanted a free choice of hospital.

People were asked if they felt they had sufficient information to make informed choices about the best provider for them (see

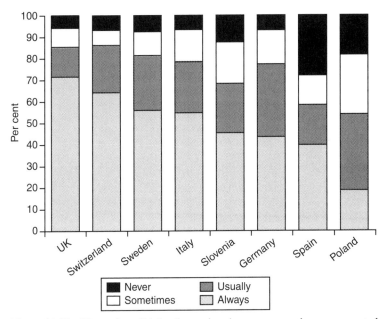

Figure 11.11   How often did the doctor involve you as much as you wanted in decisions about your care?

Table 11.11). Overall, less than half of the respondents said they had sufficient information to make an informed choice of primary care doctor, and the proportion was even less for specialist doctors and hospitals. Younger people tended to be more critical than older people of the availability of information to support provider choices and there were interesting differences between the educational groups: those with higher education were more likely than those with primary education to say they didn't have sufficient information to make informed choices (see Table 11.12).

Once again there were interesting variations between the countries (see Table 11.13). More than half the respondents in Italy were confident that they had sufficient information to choose, whereas the proportion in Spain expressing similar confidence was less than a third. It was noteworthy that in Germany and Switzerland, where free choice of specialist is currently the norm, only just over 40 per cent of respondents felt they had sufficient information to make an informed choice.

Table 11.8 Want free choice of provider (by age group)

	16–24 (n = 1267) %	25–34 (n = 1465) %	35–44 (n = 1527) %	45–54 (n = 1430) %	55–64 (n = 1150) %	65+ (n = 1280) %	Total (n = 8119) %
Primary care doctors	92	95	94	96	94	93	92
Specialist doctors	88	86	86	86	84	81	85
Hospitals	85	88	87	87	88	84	86

Table 11.9 Want free choice of provider (by educational status)

	Primary (n = 2464) %	Secondary (n = 3963) %	University (n = 1631) %
Primary care doctors	95	94	93
Specialist doctors	89	85	80
Hospitals	90	86	83

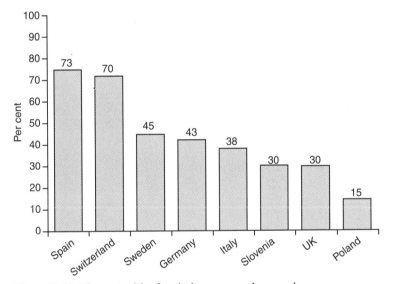

Figure 11.12   Opportunities for choice very good or good

Finally, respondents were asked to rate the extent to which patients in their country had opportunities to make choices about their health care (see Table 11.14). Younger people were much more likely to be dissatisfied with the amount of choice than older people, and people with university education were slightly more likely to be dissatisfied than those in the other two educational groups (see Table 11.15). The differences between the countries were again striking (see Figure 11.12). More than two thirds of respondents in Spain and Switzerland said they were satisfied with the opportunities for choice in their country, as against less than a third in Slovenia, the UK and Poland.

Table 11.10 Want free choice of provider (by country)

	Germany (n=1026) %	Italy (n=1021) %	Poland (n=1050) %	Slovenia (n=1014) %	Spain (n=1000) %	Sweden (n=1000) %	Switzerland (n=1000) %	UK (n=1008) %
Primary care doctors	98	86	98	98	89	86	93	87
Specialist doctors	97	83	95	87	86	31	84	79
Hospitals	94	85	94	86	78	54	85	80

Table 11.11 Those who felt they had sufficient information to choose the best provider for them (by age group)

	16–24 (n=1267) %	25–34 (n=1465) %	35–44 (n=1527) %	45–54 (n=1430) %	55–64 (n=1150) %	65+ (n=1280) %	Total (n=8119) %
Primary care doctors	39	39	42	49	53	57	**46**
Specialist doctors	31	31	32	37	41	47	**36**
Hospitals	41	38	34	41	47	49	**41**

Table 11.12 Those who felt they had sufficient information to choose the best provider for them (by educational status)

	Primary (n = 2464) %	Secondary (n = 3963) %	University (n = 1631) %
Primary care doctors	47	47	42
Specialist doctors	38	36	33
Hospitals	42	41	40

CONCLUSIONS

Our results show that the demand for an interactive communication style, more health care information and greater opportunities for involvement and choice is strong among these European patients. They expect higher standards and want to be treated more like informed consumers. They value open interpersonal communications and they want their preferences to be taken into account in decisions which affect them. In particular, people appreciate doctors who are willing to listen to what they have to say, who allow time for questions and who are able to provide comprehensible explanations. They also want more opportunities to choose providers and they require better information to facilitate this.

Doctors appear to communicate better with older people. These generational differences are especially interesting. While levels of satisfaction are still high in all age groups, younger people tend to be more dissatisfied and more critical than those who are older. This might be because their expectations are higher, or it might indicate that doctors are better at communicating with those who use health care more frequently and are hence more familiar. Certainly there was evidence that younger people want to be more actively involved in decisions about their care. Will these young people still want to be active participants when they become older or will they become more like their parents and grandparents, less critical and more content with a passive role? We cannot be certain, but it seems likely that we are witnessing a general cultural change in which people are becoming less and less content to be treated as passive recipients of health care.

The survey results also suggest that doctors are better at communicating with more educated people, perhaps because they

Table 11.13 Those who felt they had sufficient information to choose the best provider for them (by country)

	Germany (n = 1026) %	Italy (n = 1021) %	Poland (n = 1050) %	Slovenia (n = 1014) %	Spain (n = 1000) %	Sweden (n = 1000) %	Switzerland (n = 1000) %	UK (n = 1008) %
Primary care doctors	52	53	43	45	30	31	52	40
Specialist doctors	42	53	32	25	23	23	41	28
Hospitals	42	54	35	30	32	36	52	35

Table 11.14 Opportunities for patients to make health care choices (by age group)

	16–24 (n = 1267) %	25–34 (n = 1465) %	35–44 (n = 1527) %	45–54 (n = 1430) %	55–64 (n = 1150) %	65+ (n = 1280) %	Total (n = 8119) %
Very good/good	42	36	38	38	49	55	42
Moderate	42	43	41	40	33	31	39
Bad/very bad	16	21	21	22	18	14	19

Table 11.15 Opportunities for patients to make health care choices (by educational status)

	Primary *(n = 2464)* %	*Secondary* *(n = 3963)* %	*University* *(n = 1631)* %
Very good/good	41	43	42
Moderate	37	39	37
Bad/very bad	18	18	21

assume that people who are less educated do not want full information and are content with a paternalistic approach. If so, this assumption would appear to be misplaced; the need for information and understanding about health issues was apparent in all educational groups. People who are less articulate or less confident in their dealings with health professionals do not necessarily want less information and involvement.

Doctors, especially GPs, are still seen as the primary source of information about diseases and treatments, but increasing numbers of people also seek health information from other sources. Many people said they found it difficult to access reliable information. This inhibits their ability to make informed choices about new treatments or about who to consult or which hospital they should go to. This problem was not confined to those in the lower educational groups: the higher the educational level, the more likely people were to express dissatisfaction with the availability of information.

The internet has not yet made a very significant impact on people's knowledge about new treatments. The situation may change rapidly, but it will be important to develop reliable public websites and portals which meet patients' needs for balanced and trustworthy information on the full range of treatment options for a given condition. If these are not available there is a risk that commercially-sponsored websites selling inappropriate or 'quack' remedies will distort the demand for new treatments. It will also be important to take steps to ensure that this information is accessible to all sections of society, not just those who are better educated or those who have ready access to the internet at home.

As people throughout Europe become more educated and better informed, it seems likely that tolerance of a paternalistic style of health care delivery will diminish even further. People will refuse to accept that 'doctor knows best', preferring to make their own decisions whenever possible. Patients of the future will expect to play an active part in managing their own care and in treatment decisions; they will be better informed and they will expect to be offered choices.

These trends were apparent in all our study countries, but there was evidence that the gap between public expectations and the reality of health care delivery is greater in some countries than others. The reasons for this are likely to be complex. Except at the extremes, there were no obvious relationships between characteristics of the health system and the level of responsiveness to patients' needs in terms of resource levels, funding source or organization. The mode of funding (taxation or social insurance) could not account for the differences between the countries, nor did factors such as the level of decentralization, the extent to which patients are expected to make out-of-pocket payments or the existence of a primary care gatekeeping system. It was certainly true that the highest spending country, Switzerland, achieved better results in terms of responsiveness to patients than Poland, which has the least well resourced health system among our study countries. But patients in Germany, another high spender on health care, seemed less satisfied with doctor-patient communications than those in the UK and Sweden, where spending levels are considerably lower.

There was evidence that patients' expectations of involvement in decisions about their care differed between the countries, with people in Spain and Poland exhibiting a greater preference for a paternalistic style than those in Switzerland and Germany. But dissatisfaction with involvement in treatment decisions was also high in Spain and Poland, suggesting that opinions are divided in these countries.

Overall, a picture emerges of generally high levels of satisfaction with health professionals' communication skills in countries like Switzerland, Sweden and the UK, while patients in Poland, Italy and Germany are more dissatisfied. Levels of dissatisfaction in Germany were surprising given that Germans use health services more frequently than people in the other countries. Polish patients seem to experience considerably more communication problems than those in the other countries. The family doctor service in Poland is relatively new, so the negative assessments of Polish respondents may reflect early teething problems with the new system. Paradoxically, in Italy patients' reports of doctors' communication skills were relatively positive, but the proportion that rated communication as good was low, suggesting higher expectations and greater dissatisfaction among Italian patients. In these countries there seems to be a serious mismatch between the way in which doctors and other health care providers communicate and what many patients want or expect. It seems that public attitudes are changing faster than health professionals realize and the gulf between what people want and the way in which health care is delivered is widening.

Expectations of more information, more involvement and more choice are rising everywhere, especially among younger, more educated people. The overwhelming majority of respondents wanted to be able to choose their health care providers, but only in Spain and Switzerland were the majority satisfied with the opportunities for choice; more than half of those in the other countries were dissatisfied. The demand for choice of provider was exceptionally high everywhere except Sweden. It is not entirely clear why the results from Sweden were so different, but they may be a reflection of the recent political debate about privatization. Swedish people tend to go to hospitals administered by their local county council rather than further afield, and perhaps people are content with this restriction. However, completely free choice of specialist or hospital is fairly uncommon in the other countries too. People are not used to choice in health care, yet most seem to want more of it. This is especially true in countries such as Slovenia, Poland and the UK, where opportunities for choice have been particularly limited to date.

The slightly lower enthusiasm for choice among those with university education was interesting. Perhaps this is indicative of increased understanding of the disadvantages of free choice, or due to greater awareness of the limited available information to support informed choice. Nevertheless, even in this group the demand for more choice was high.

People increasingly want information and support to make their own informed choices of providers and treatments. Services must adapt to accommodate a more consumerist approach to health care utilization. Investment in accessible, reliable and user-friendly information about diseases, treatments and indicators of the quality of care offered by different providers is urgently needed to ensure that public support for health systems is maintained.

NOTE

1 Degner, L.F., Sloan, J.A. and Venkatesh, P. (1997) The Control Preferences Scale, *Canadian Journal of Nursing Research*, 29: 21–43.

12

KEY ISSUES FOR EUROPEAN PATIENTS

STRENGTHS AND WEAKNESSES OF HEALTH SYSTEMS

Responsiveness

Health care is very important to, and highly valued by, the public in each of the eight countries where we carried out our research. In many cases it attracts more support than any other public service and reported satisfaction levels are generally high. However, levels of satisfaction are affected by expectations, which in turn are influenced by cultural factors and experience, so high satisfaction ratings do not tell the whole story. It was clear from our research that satisfaction with the system and the way it is organized and funded can, and often does, coexist with particular concerns about quality and access. It was also apparent that people who have had satisfactory experiences themselves, particularly those with recent experience of health care, tended to express greater satisfaction with the health system as a whole than those whose personal experience was less positive or less recent.

Younger people tend to be more likely to voice criticisms than older people. This could be because they are lower users of the health care system and therefore less familiar with its strengths, or it might indicate higher expectations and less tolerance of its failings. If this tendency among younger people is indicative of future trends in expectations, health policy makers must take note because there is a risk that public support for the way health care is organized and delivered may begin to erode. Many people in our focus groups were pessimistic about the future prospects for health care in their country and concerned that the system would not be able to provide them with the best possible treatment when they needed it.

The experience of illness is highly personal and the need for sympathetic and humane treatment is especially strong when one is ill. Levels of satisfaction with primary care were high and most people also expressed confidence in specialist and hospital care, but there were concerns that the personal touch is being squeezed out. People complained of being treated more as a number than a person and many were concerned about complexity and discontinuities in care. Technical skill and efficiency is valued highly, but people also set great store by good interpersonal relations with health professionals. For the most part these are good, but participants also pointed to many failures. Our study provided evidence that much good practice exists, but it is by no means universal. There are still considerable gaps between what European patients want and what is currently available, and these gaps will widen unless health systems can adapt to changes in public expectations.

Access

Problems with waiting times and access arrangements were by far the most commonly voiced complaint in our focus groups. Having to wait for advice or treatment that the patient perceives to be necessary and possibly urgent is a particularly depressing and disempowering experience. People in six of the eight countries complained of having to wait days, weeks and even months for appointments with health professionals and many talked of long hours spent sitting in clinics waiting to see a doctor. The two exceptions were Germany and Switzerland, where generous funding and staffing levels have meant that patients experience few problems in accessing the help they need at times convenient to them.

Waiting was perceived to be a serious problem everywhere else, albeit to varying degrees. People in Italy, Poland and Slovenia complained about long waits for certain services. Access problems were perceived to be on the increase in Sweden and there were fears that staff recruitment difficulties would make the situation even worse in the future. In Spain there was a sense that the system was too bound up in red tape, causing problems with getting appointments to see doctors. In the UK there was a high level of concern about waiting times. Patients complained of feeling frustrated and disempowered because their time was viewed as expendable by staff and by the system. Having to wait also induces anxiety in patients concerned about the consequences for their health.

Authorities in several countries have made various attempts to reduce waiting times, but the problem has proved fairly intractable. For example, in Sweden minimum waiting time guarantees for specific services were dropped when they proved impossible to implement. When access to primary care is perceived to be difficult, patients tend to go to open access clinics such as hospital emergency departments or walk-in centres, where they are likely to have to queue for some time. When the waiting time to access GPs in Spain was reduced by 10 per cent, use of emergency services dropped by 20 per cent, underscoring the need for a 'whole system' approach to tackling access problems. In Italy and Poland some people admitted to making use of personal contacts to help them bypass the queues. These 'informal channels' include doctor friends who can help pull strings to speed up access to specialists, and in some cases illegal payments or bribes were reported. In Slovenia and the UK some successful initiatives have resulted in reduced waits and made a noticeable difference to some patients, but the overall sense is of a problem that just won't go away without increasing spending to unaffordable levels. This has led governments to introduce various restrictions on access as a means of controlling demand.

The introduction of gatekeeping systems, whereby patients cannot access specialist care without a referral from a GP, is one such measure. In Poland, where such a system has recently been introduced, the establishment of a family doctor system was widely welcomed but there were concerns about the new restrictions on access to specialists. In particular, some parents wanted to retain the freedom to consult paediatricians about their children's health. Likewise in Slovenia patients valued the easier and less formal interaction they could have with GPs, but they were concerned that access to certain services (e.g. laboratory tests) was more restricted than previously.

In Germany and Switzerland, where people are used to having free access to specialists, attempts to introduce voluntary gatekeeping systems are meeting some resistance. On the other hand, people in the UK who have had long experience of such a system seem to accept and value it, although some focus group participants said they would welcome the opportunity for greater flexibility, including direct access to certain specialists. In general it seems that willingness to accept a more restricted referral system depends in large part on public confidence in primary care. If that is seen as offering fast, flexible access to high quality care, then most patients are willing to be guided by their GP's opinion on whether they need specialist attention.

Many of the policy initiatives examined in our study are linked to attempts to solve the access problem. For example, nurses and pharmacists are being encouraged to take on extended roles to allow doctors to spend more time on tasks which require their specific skills; telephone helplines and email consultations are intended to speed up access to health advice, avoiding the need for face-to-face contact; information and support for patients in self-care and self-management of chronic disease may help to reduce demand; and the various attempts to encourage patients to exercise choice are intended to inject competition into health systems in the hope that this will foster greater productivity and efficiency.

Equity

Equity of access according to need is a defining principle of European health systems and it continues to command popular support. Geographical differences in the availability and quality of care were considered unacceptable. Many participants in our research felt it was the responsibility of government to reduce regional inequalities in the quality and delivery of services. Geographical variations in the distribution and quality of services are common. For example, in Italy there was a strong sense that services were better in the north of the country than in the south or central areas, and in Poland and Slovenia there were concerns about the concentration of doctors and services in the urban areas, with rural areas being relatively deprived.

There were a few signs that traditional support for universal equitable coverage was wavering in the face of a rise in consumerist attitudes. For example, most focus group participants in Germany expressed strong support for the solidarity principle on which the insurance system is based, but a few questioned whether contribution-free family health insurance should be maintained – for example, for non-working wives. Attitudes were mixed, however, and conflicting views were commonplace. For example, some participants in Slovenia felt that people who indulged in dangerous sporting activities should be required to pay higher insurance premiums, but others argued strongly in support of equal access for all.

Pessimism about the financial basis of the health care systems was widespread and there was a sense that current levels of coverage were unsustainable in the longer term. Many people feared they would have to pay extra charges or save to cover their health care needs in old age. People were particularly concerned to avoid what they saw as the American problem – a 'two-tier' system with good quality health care for those who can afford it and only basic, second-rate services for the rest.

Co-payments for medicines and other services and 'top-up' insurance schemes are common and the extent to which patients are expected to make out-of-pocket contributions is increasing. Public concern about direct payment issues was apparent in all eight countries, in particular those where health care funding comes from social insurance. For example, German patients complained about the introduction of direct charges for certain diagnostic and therapeutic procedures and the high cost of supplementary insurance; Polish patients were conscious of having to pay significantly more for their medicines; and in Switzerland there was considerable concern about rising premiums. Patients in the UK were concerned about rising prescription and dental charges, but because health care is funded out of central taxation they were much less aware of the costs than people in the countries where insurees receive bills and have to make claims for the care they have received.

Most participants in our research saw increased dependence on out-of-pocket payments as an unwelcome but inevitable trend. Many people voiced strong objections to user charges on grounds of equity. Co-payments were seen as placing an unacceptably heavy burden on poorer people and those who are less healthy, but some people (e.g. younger people in Italy, and wealthier city dwellers in Poland and Spain) supported the principle of charging for specific services. Some Spanish people felt charges for accommodation while in hospital would be acceptable. Others (e.g. some Swedish people) felt that a certain level of direct charges might be acceptable if they were restricted to those who led unhealthy lifestyles (e.g. smokers) or those who wanted to take medicines of dubious efficacy. However, many participants expressed the view that paying just to speed up access – queue-jumping in other words – was unacceptable.

Despite their concerns about equity, many people were tolerant of the coexistence of public and private systems. In Spain support for state-funded health care is strong, but a substantial minority defend the coexistence of public and private systems. In Italy the existence of a relatively large private sector was seen as offering an opportunity for choice, rather than a wasteful duplication. Problems with accessing care in the public systems provide the major incentive for using private services. For example, people in the southern and central regions of Italy, where health care is perceived to be of lower quality than in the north, expressed the view that you have to pay to get better care. In Poland many people believe that private health centres provide better care, but there are also concerns about the unfairness of a system which benefits those who are better off.

The public commitment to equity in health care is complex. Although most participants in our research voiced strong beliefs in the principle of equity, and they were particularly concerned about socioeconomic and geographical inequalities in access to care, many were prepared to tolerate the existence of a private sector for those who could afford to pay more. A few people questioned the solidarity principle, seeing some groups as more deserving of collectively-funded provision than others. However, we did not find any evidence to suggest that these uncertainties about the moral basis of collective health care provision are becoming more prevalent. On the contrary, belief in access to all according to need rather than the ability to pay continues to be a defining principle of the health systems in these European countries.

NEW PROFESSIONAL ROLES

Doctors

Doctors are trusted and very highly regarded in all eight countries. Family doctors are expected to provide medical care and diagnoses, but also psychological and social support. For example, Italian patients stressed the importance of the 'physician-psychologist' role, with family doctors acting as friend and confidante. But doctors' medical knowledge and technical competence was also seen as very important. Doctor-patient communication was considered to be the most important indicator of good health care. Our survey results indicate that this aspect of health care is handled relatively well in most cases and the majority of patients were satisfied with doctors' communication skills, but there is clearly room for improvement. For example, German participants said doctors should talk to patients more and prescribe less. Italian patients complained that doctors' manner was sometimes distant and detached and they were unwilling to explain illnesses, treatments or hospital procedures. Complaints that doctors have too little time for patients because they are overburdened with bureaucratic responsibilities were common.

Participants were particularly critical of doctors who seemed to put financial concerns before the interests of their patients. For example, German participants felt some doctors had got the balance wrong between their business and financial interests and their health care responsibilities, and there were complaints from people in Poland and Slovenia that doctors sometimes charged patients for services that should be provided free at the point of use.

Continuity

Initial reactions to the suggestion that waiting times could be reduced if patients were willing to see health professionals other than their own family doctor were largely negative. Most were unwilling to sacrifice the continuing personal relationship which is still highly valued, especially by older people. For example, Swedish participants feared that consulting unfamiliar doctors would put the onus on them to remember and repeat details of their medical history, thus increasing the possibility of error. They also felt such a system would result in contradictory advice from different practitioners.

However, younger people in some countries were more willing to contemplate seeing different doctors. This may be because of the different nature of health problems experienced by younger people or it may indicate that attitudes are changing. A few participants in Sweden remarked that the relationship with their doctor was so impersonal already that it would make little difference. Younger people in the UK were also quite willing to trade continuity for quick access. This may be a result of greater experience in these countries of group practice in primary care. For example, general practices in the UK are larger nowadays, with four to six (and sometimes more) GPs working together in partnership. Many offer patients the option of seeing any doctor in the practice rather than just the one they are registered with, and some patients are happy to do this in the knowledge that each doctor can access their medical record and therefore has some knowledge of their history. The sense of continuity is preserved by the familiarity of the surroundings and the existence of a good record system.

The opportunity to consult unidentified doctors or nurses on unfamiliar territory was not generally welcomed, except for emergency care. High rates of use of hospital accident and emergency departments is evidence of people's willingness to consult strangers in emergency situations, but this does not apply in continuing care. The familiarity of a local clinic or health centre and a continuous relationship with a single doctor who knows a patient's medical history was generally viewed as even more important than fast access to medical advice. But people were willing to concede that walk-in centres could have a valuable role in treating minor injuries and other acute problems and could be especially useful for commuters or those whose working hours make it difficult to access their local family doctor's clinic at convenient times.

Nurses

Participants in the focus groups had mixed views on whether nurses should take on extended roles. For example, in Poland nurses were highly valued for their personal approach, friendliness, skill, efficiency and ready availability, but many people felt they were not sufficiently well trained to take on a more responsible role. Men and women tended to express different views and these were often mediated by their previous experience of nursing care. Men with little experience of receiving care from nurses saw them as doctor's assistants only. Those men who had more recent experience of nursing care tended to resist the idea that nurses should take on more responsibilities because they saw them as overburdened enough already. They were less concerned about enhancing nurses' professional autonomy and more concerned that nurses shouldn't be burdened with responsibilities doctors don't want. On the other hand, women tended to feel that there were some situations – for example, midwifery, where nurses had more authority than doctors and this should be officially recognized.

Similar debates took place in focus groups in the other countries, with similar differences between male and female participants. For example, Swedish participants had great confidence in nurses and younger women expressed the view that they should be given more responsibility, but young men tended to think the existing balance was about right. Participants in the UK who had experienced care from nurse practitioners undertaking extended responsibilities were comfortable with this development, but there was a strong feeling that nurses should not be overburdened or poorly rewarded for taking on more work. On the other hand, people in Italy, Slovenia and Spain tended to cling to the notion that the nurse's principal role was to provide practical support to the doctor, with no independent role in diagnosis or therapy.

Nurses were seen as easier to talk to than doctors, and as attentive, caring and closer to the patient. They were felt to have an important role in providing patients with supplementary information and reassurance, softening the medical setting and offering support in distressing situations. Some people could see financial advantages in giving nurses an extended role, but they were concerned about clinical responsibility and liability issues. Most people believed that prescribing should remain the doctor's responsibility, except for very limited indications, and all groups stressed the need for more training for nurses if they were to take on a wider role.

Pharmacists

Many people use pharmacists as their first port of call when suffering minor ailments and there was widespread recognition of pharmacists' specific knowledge and experience. For example, people in Slovenia saw them as having the most up-to-date knowledge about new medicines, frequently better than doctors. Participants in Germany remarked that they were excellent information providers – customer-oriented professionals who are good at talking the language of patients. They also provide an important safety function in checking that the doctor's prescription is correct.

The growing market in over-the-counter medicines is testimony to the public's reliance on pharmacists' advice and the products they sell. But views on whether they should take on more direct responsibility for prescribing were largely negative. Their role was seen as complementary to that of doctors, but not as a substitute. Some people saw them primarily as shopkeepers running small businesses, while others saw them as highly trained health professionals, but there was some concern about potential conflicts of interest between these two roles.

In general our findings suggest that European patients tend to react conservatively to suggestions that professional roles might change, but they readily adapt to these changes when they occur. As long as people are reassured that staff are adequately trained and rewarded for the roles they take on, they will accept and indeed embrace the changes in the long run.

REMOTE ACCESS TO HEALTH ADVICE

Telephone

In some countries patients are encouraged to phone their own doctor for advice as an alternative to a clinic visit. This facility was generally welcomed, although Swedish participants pointed out that the telephone demands good verbal skills which could be a problem for some people, particularly the elderly. In Slovenia patients are supposed to be able to get advice from their GPs over the phone, but practice varies a lot. Some doctors complain that they aren't reimbursed for giving telephone advice. Some participants in the Slovenian focus groups were concerned that responding to calls could interfere with the doctor's work in the clinic, distracting attention from their other patients.

People in the UK who had used NHS Direct, the new national telephone helpline run by nurses, were very positive about this development, although not everyone was aware of it. Parents, in particular, valued the opportunity to access quick advice when their children are ill and people saw that it could help reduce the burden on hospitals and health centres. Those who had not used it or were unaware of its existence were more cautious. They felt the telephone would not be appropriate for complex consultations. Symptoms might be missed or misinterpreted and the anonymity of the person at the other end of the phone line was seen as a drawback. How could they be sure they were speaking to a genuine health professional? People were also concerned about how they would seek redress if they received bad advice.

Similar concerns were expressed by focus group participants in the other countries. Experience of using telephone helplines was limited, however. Some German health insurance agencies are establishing systems similar to the British one and commercial providers are coming into this market in a number of countries, but few participants had used these services. People felt they could be very useful for minor problems or for guidance on administrative issues, but the telephone was seen as too prone to the risk of misdiagnosis to be of much use in more serious cases. Participants in all countries tended to place great stress on the importance of face-to-face contact, direct observation and hands-on examination. The relative anonymity of the telephone was seen as having advantages in certain situations and the opportunity to access advice on minor problems without bothering the doctor was welcomed. But people were reluctant to contemplate its use as a substitute for face-to-face contact when they were seriously concerned about their symptoms.

Telemedicine

Telemedicine does not yet play a significant role in the provision of health care in any of our study countries and none of the focus group participants had direct experience of it. Most people saw it as being more relevant for doctor-to-doctor consultation – for example, GPs seeking specialist advice, than for direct patient-to-doctor contact. Many were sceptical about the prospect of telemedicine being used to diagnose or treat patients. For example, people in Poland and Spain believed strongly in the importance of physical examination and detailed knowledge of the patient's medical history and they could not see how remote consultations using telemedicine could replace these fundamental aspects of person-to-person contact. Participants in the UK felt it might have diagnostic relevance in certain cases (e.g. for skin conditions where visual identification of symptoms might be possible) but they were sceptical about its use in other situations.

Some people could see potential advantages for those living in rural areas who could not easily access advice from the best specialists. German participants felt it might facilitate international consultations, although remote diagnosis without direct physical contact is not yet permitted in Germany. Younger participants in the Italian focus groups, particularly men, were quite enthusiastic about the possibility of using telemedicine to gain access to famous specialists, but female participants saw it as too cold and detached. Swiss participants were prepared to contemplate long-distance counselling, but they weren't prepared to put themselves into the hands of a 'digital doctor' for long-distance treatment. Some British participants were concerned about the possibility of abuse – for example, circulation of the images on the internet.

Here once again we can see the predictable pattern of a conservative response to these innovations from those who had never used them, but cautious optimism from the few who had relevant experience. Experience of telephone helplines and telemedicine is very limited at present. Concerns have been raised about the cost-effectiveness of these developments, but they may prove to be an efficient way of addressing people's expressed needs for quick advice on a wide range of problems. The extent to which they will act as a substitute for existing modes of access is more doubtful however. Perhaps their impact should be measured in terms of whether they address previously unmet needs, rather than whether they reduce demand for other services.

REGULATING TESTS AND TREATMENTS

Complementary therapies

Complementary medicine is growing in popularity in all the study countries, but the extent to which it is officially recognized and supported varies widely. For example, in Germany many conventional practitioners offer complementary therapies in addition to orthodox ones and some of these are reimbursable by the insurance schemes. Similarly in Switzerland there is official acknowledgement of the role of complementary medicine and several therapies are reimbursed by insurance. A federal government office is considering how best to evaluate the clinical and cost-effectiveness of complementary therapies. A similar initiative is underway in the UK under the auspices of the NHS research and development programme. British GPs are increasingly recommending, endorsing and even providing complementary therapies alongside other treatments. The market for complementary therapies is also steadily increasing in Sweden and there is now an official classification system which groups the different therapies according to whether they are approved natural remedies, remedies awaiting approval or remedies that do not have official status.

However, there is still a lot of resistance to complementary medicine, in particular in Italy, Spain and Slovenia, especially from doctors. Use of complementary therapies appears to be especially low in Italy and Spain and there is no official recognition or regulation of alternative practitioners. Some therapies are considered more acceptable than others. For example, various types of manipulation therapy, such as chiropractic therapy or osteopathy, are now accepted as standard treatments in some places, whereas there is more scepticism about the value of treatments like acupuncture, herbalism or reflexology.

In most cases complementary therapies are used alongside orthodox treatments, rather than as a substitute. The typical user of complementary medicine tends to be a young or middle-aged female, well-educated and health-conscious. Nurses and younger doctors tend to be more positive about alternative treatment approaches than older doctors and the leaders of the medical profession still largely resist these developments. There are exceptions, however. In some parts of Europe (e.g. Germany, Switzerland and Slovenia) health spas have been popular for many years and in certain cases, especially in German-speaking countries, they are a well-accepted part of rehabilitation with the cost of a stay at a health spa being reclaimable from health insurers.

Focus group participants' views of complementary medicine were mixed, with both enthusiasm and scepticism reflected in people's comments. Some people felt these therapies were more 'natural' and therefore less harmful, but others were concerned about unproven therapies and unregulated, bogus practitioners. In several countries there are plans to extend existing regulatory systems to include complementary practitioners. This may change the nature of complementary medicine, possibly reducing its attractiveness to its adherents.

The enthusiasm for complementary medicine is a powerful demonstration of people's desire to help themselves, as well as an indication of their frustration with the limitations of orthodox medicine. If it is externally regulated and integrated with orthodox medicine, it is likely that complementary medicine will become an addition to the therapeutic armamentarium of orthodox practitioners, who will then control access to it. This may enhance its acceptability to the medical profession, especially if such treatments pass the efficacy test, but it could reduce its distinctiveness, and hence its appeal, to patients. Whatever happens, the pressure from the public to include complementary therapies in the list of reimbursable treatments seems likely to continue.

Rationing medicines

Authorities in some of our study countries have introduced limited drug lists, restricting reimbursement to medicines that can pass tests of cost-effectiveness. The basis for these restrictions is not widely understood by members of the public and several participants complained about them. For example, Swiss people were concerned about rising premiums but were not willing to accept restrictions on services to reduce costs. Many people in Germany expressed the view that resources are used inefficiently and there is considerable waste in the health care system. Several participants felt there was scope to increase efficiency and a few felt that greater effort should be made to control the number of doctors. However, there was little evidence that people were fully cognizant of mechanisms for setting priorities in health care, and with the exception of Sweden there have been few attempts to engage members of the public in the process.

There was some discussion and debate in the focus groups about whether new medicines to treat previously untreatable conditions, such as obesity, baldness or impotence, should be reimbursed. Considerable effort has been made by the authorities in Sweden to engage the public in decisions about priorities. Swedes now tend to accept that there is a need to set limits on expenditure and that priority-setting is inevitable. Preparations such as *Viagra* and *Xenical* were originally reimbursed in Sweden, but a government decision in April 2001 to cut the subsidy to bring the rules into harmony with many other European countries was largely supported by the Swedish public. However, about a third of young people thought that financial support for the cost of anti-impotence treatments should continue.

Public debate about rationing has been more muted in most of the other countries. In Italy there is growing awareness of the need to weigh the balance of cost, benefit and harm in relation to new treatments, but people don't approve of any restrictions that amount to discrimination against specific user groups. In Switzerland, with its tradition of direct democracy, there is a recognition that the debate about rationing must take place openly and publicly and any decisions should arise from societal consensus, in line with Swiss tradition. In England, the Department of Health is establishing a Citizen's Council to provide guidance on the values underpinning judgements about whether particular treatments should be recommended for use.

Politicians in most countries have been very reluctant to enter the debate about rationing, but there is growing acceptance of the idea that it will simply not be possible to pay for every conceivable medical intervention out of public funds, and priorities have to be set. If that is to be done rationally and fairly, the public must be engaged in helping to decide how priorities should be determined and which values should prevail.

Genomics

Another topic which has been the subject of considerable public debate is the new developments in genomics. Participants in our focus groups reflected the variety of opinions and arguments for and against genetic screening. For example, in Switzerland, German-speaking men were more receptive to genetic tests than women and French speakers, who tended to see tests to measure the risk of falling ill in the future as a step too far. Spanish people were wary of the latest scientific breakthroughs and were particularly concerned about the possibility of human cloning. However, one in four

Spaniards complain that they cannot access the most modern medical technologies and about half see genetic tests as acceptable. Participants in the Polish focus groups tended to reject the strictures of the Catholic Church which is opposed to prenatal testing, but they were concerned about the psychological impact of early diagnosis, especially if people had to live with the knowledge that they were at high risk but there was little they could do about it.

Survey evidence suggests that many Italians have high expectations of biotechnologies, believing that genetic research will eventually make it possible to defeat serious diseases. Nevertheless, some of the participants in the Italian focus groups said they would rather not know about the likelihood of developing disease in the future, preferring to adopt a fatalistic approach – what will be will be. Participants in Slovenia thought genetic screening would be acceptable only if effective therapies were available to treat any diseases identified. Only younger women thought it would be advantageous to know about predisposition to particular illnesses. This pattern was reflected in the British focus groups, where parents of young children were more likely to be positive about prenatal screening for abnormalities. While the majority view was that genetic developments can be useful, some felt this amounted to unacceptable tampering with nature.

Concern was expressed in a number of groups about who should have access to the results of diagnostic or genetic screening tests. For example, German participants were worried about adverse consequences if this information got into the hands of employers or insurance agencies. Most people felt such tests should only be undergone following medical advice and there was concern about the increasing availability of self-diagnosis testing kits which can be bought from high street pharmacies. British participants felt there was a risk of creating a nation of hypochondriacs if everyone could diagnose themselves.

Europeans are by no means starry-eyed about the prospects of medical advance following the knowledge breakthroughs in genomics. People can see both the pros and cons of greater access to genetic screening and views range from cautious optimism to concern about the negative effects. Most people make a connection between screening and the availability of effective treatments or preventive strategies, and on the whole they don't want one without the other.

PROMOTING PATIENT AUTONOMY

Health information

More information about health, illness, treatments and sources of help was a clearly expressed demand in all our study countries. For example, Polish patients wanted more information about how to navigate their way through the reformed health system, how to choose a GP, access a specialist and claim health insurance. They also wanted detailed information on diagnostic tests and treatment options, risks, benefits, side-effects and costs, including the availability and cost of complementary medicines. And they wanted to know how to look after themselves following medical treatment or inpatient admission, including advice on diet, activity and exercise and what to do about symptoms and relapses. Our survey results suggest that this need for information is largely unmet in Poland at present and only partially met in most of the other countries.

Our survey showed that people increasingly want information to enable them to make informed choices about treatments or about which health care provider to consult. These needs were echoed and amplified in the focus groups. For example, participants in Germany felt reasonably well-informed about illness and prevention, but they lacked information about the quality of hospitals and ambulatory care, the technical skills and special interests of GPs and specialists, and where to find independent sources of advice and assistance, such as ombudspersons or patient counsellors.

The Swedish research identified an apparently insatiable demand for information, especially among younger and better-educated people and those with poorer health. People want to understand what's happening to them and to feel more in control of their care, and information is seen as the key to this. However, some Swedish participants admitted to sometimes holding back from asking questions of health professionals for fear of appearing stupid or too demanding. They also complained about doctors who gave them too little time or used language they did not understand.

Women tend to be more active information-seekers than men and younger, middle-class people are especially likely to seek out independent sources of information and advice. People with chronic illnesses and parents with children at home often go to considerable lengths to obtain information from a variety of sources. Nevertheless, doctors are still by far and away the most popular source of information. Most people trust their doctors, but they are often frustrated by the limited information they provide so they seek additional information to supplement, and sometimes to check, their doctor's advice. Younger people are more likely than older people to question the advice they are given by health professionals and less likely to believe that 'doctor knows best'.

It was clear from our research that people used and trusted information differently depending on whether they wanted to satisfy a need or a curiosity. For example, for Italian patients with a newly-diagnosed illness the most reliable and trustworthy sources were the family doctor, relatives and friends. They relied on the doctor for advice about the disease, clinical tests and how to prepare for them, and for information about therapies and drug side-effects. But friends and relatives were consulted for advice on the best doctors and health centres and how to access them. Participants also reported that exchange of experiences with other patients or ex-patients is the most reassuring and efficient way to get information. Advice in magazines and on TV programmes was seen as less trust-worthy by participants in the Italian focus groups, not very credible, contradictory and in some cases even dangerous, and too concerned with commercial interests and ratings, or dictated by the latest fashion trends. Interestingly, this scepticism was reflected in the survey results: people in Italy and Spain were least likely to see the mass media as a source of information about new treatments while substantial minorities in the other countries did look to newspapers, magazines or broadcast media for useful health information.

The internet

There is a proliferation of health websites in various languages. Many of these are commercially sponsored, but national authorities and health care providers in many countries have developed websites to provide public information on health issues. For example, in Slovenia the National Health Information Clearing House is being developed to offer access to medical and other health data, initially for health professionals but eventually for patients as well. It is anticipated that patients will be able to get information on local waiting lists, availability of specialists and the quality of health care providers. In the UK, NHS Direct Online and the National Electronic Library for Health provide publicly-accessible information on a wide variety of health topics together with links to a large number of quality-assessed websites developed by other providers. And in Poland a project sponsored by the European Commission is providing internet cafes in health centres and clinics to help people access health information and advice on prevention.

Our telephone survey demonstrated that the internet is still relatively insignificant as a source of health information for European patients. For example, only 10 per cent of respondents saw it as a source of information about new treatments. But this figure masks considerable variation between countries, between age groups and between people with different levels of education. The proportion who sought health information from the internet rose to more than 15 per cent in Sweden, Switzerland and the UK and nearly one in five people with a university degree saw the internet as a useful source of information. Its significance seems likely to grow dramatically over the next few years, but until internet access is universal there is a risk that it will exacerbate differences between those who are 'information rich' and those who are 'information poor'.

Focus group participants reported various problems with using the internet to find health information. They welcomed the opportunity it gives for quick access to information from anywhere in the world, but many said they found the quantity of websites overwhelming and finding reliable information could take considerable time and effort. Others complained of difficulties in evaluating the quality of information on health websites and many were suspicious of their reliability and trustworthiness. There were calls for a trustworthy gateway to quality-controlled sites to help people through the maze.

Some websites offer the facility to consult a health professional for advice by email. Attitudes to online consultations were mixed. Many Italians saw this as an important additional benefit of internet access, but people in Spain were more sceptical. They were concerned about the possibility of errors and misinterpretation. To avoid these risks they felt 'virtual' consultations should only take place if the doctor at the other end of the line was familiar with the patient's history, and they should be restricted to minor problems only. Many older people were unwilling to contemplate the idea of online consultations. For them, the presence of a doctor was essential and the internet was described as 'cold' in contrast to the 'warmth' of personal contact. Some UK participants were concerned about the difficulties they might face in composing and understanding email communications. They were not confident about their writing skills and they feared they wouldn't be able to decipher medical terms. Email was seen as more anonymous than the telephone, and people were uncertain about the credentials of online doctors. They were also concerned that email advice might be slow. But the advantages of anonymity were also recognized and younger people in particular were positive about the opportunities it could offer for getting a second opinion. The demand for email consultations seems likely to increase. Strategies will have to be developed to cope with this demand and to enable people to judge the quality of the information provided.

Self-diagnosis, self-medication, self-care

Most Europeans are reasonably confident about caring for themselves when they have minor illnesses. Much health care takes place in the home, with families and friends the primary source of advice. The local pharmacy is often the first port of call if a need for bio-chemical remedies has been identified. Self-medication is common and sales of over-the-counter medicines are increasing everywhere. Most of these remedies are relatively harmless and people usually use them responsibly, but in Spain there was some concern about bacterial resistance associated with self-medicated antibiotics, despite their official 'prescription-only' status.

Most people recognize the need to take responsibility for their own health, although ideas vary about what this means. For example, in discussing the issue of responsibility some Swedish participants emphasized the need to keep medical appointments and take prescribed medicines as directed, whereas others felt it meant being aware of behavioural risks, adopting a healthy lifestyle, giving up smoking, going to the gym, providing information to the doctor, participating actively in treatment decisions and doing everything possible to manage disease themselves. A similar range of views was evident in the focus group discussions in other countries, with some adopting the more restricted view that responsibility simply meant following doctors' instructions, while others saw it as taking charge of their own health and health care wherever possible. Some participants with chronic diseases had experience of active monitoring and self-management of their condition – for example monitoring blood pressure or testing their blood glucose or cholesterol level, but others found the idea of self-management somewhat alien.

Self-help groups exist in all the study countries. In Germany, health insurance agencies are required to provide financial support for patient groups and there are also many professional self-help and advice facilities sponsored by local authorities or charities. Many patient groups in Slovenia have developed journals and websites to communicate with their members and the wider public. Self-help groups are a relatively recent phenomenon in Spain and they are patchily distributed. Some groups, for example those for AIDS, cancer or multiple sclerosis, are professionally organized, while others depend on voluntary participation of patients or their relatives. In Switzerland and in many of the other countries a national umbrella body exists to direct the public to appropriate self-help groups and to coordinate their activities.

Involvement in treatment decisions

Our survey reinforced the sense that a more paternalistic view of the doctor-patient relationship prevails in Poland and Spain, among patients as well as doctors, than in the other study countries. In countries like Germany, Italy, Sweden, Switzerland and the UK, patients are becoming more self-confident, particularly younger ones, and increasingly they want to play a more active role in their medical care. They want to be given information about treatment options and outcomes and to be involved in decisions. Governments in Sweden and the UK are taking a lead in persuading health professionals to involve patients in clinical decision making. Rights to second opinions are being reinforced in several countries. In Switzerland there have been several campaigns to promote patient empowerment and to encourage a more questioning approach to medical advice. Our survey results suggest these initiatives may now be having an effect, but providers have been slow to respond by giving active support for patient education, involvement and choice.

Paternalistic attitudes still prevail in many quarters. Many patients are disappointed when doctors don't take account of their preferences, or when they resist their attempts to get involved or take more control. Participants in the UK complained that the way care is delivered tends to undermine their sense of control and self-reliance. The obvious pressures on staff struggling with heavy workloads made patients reluctant to make demands for fear of being labelled difficult. Italian participants said they were afraid they might appear arrogant and presumptuous if they questioned the doctor's authority. German participants pointed out that it takes a lot of commitment to take more control, especially when faced with professional hostility to the idea. Most patients are aware of the constraints on staff and restrict their demands accordingly. Many voluntarily ration their time in consultations, conscious of doctors' busy workloads and the large numbers of people waiting to see them, but this tends to mask the desire for greater involvement, with the result that professionals assume it is not wanted.

Electronic patient-held records

The medical smart card was the most popular of the future scenarios presented to the focus groups. Smart cards are already in use as an administrative tool in Germany and Slovenia where they are used to register people's insurance status. The focus groups were asked to consider their reactions to using a card that contained comprehensive medical records which they could use when consulting different health professionals.

Most people welcomed the idea, seeing it as a concrete solution to a deeply-felt problem. Italian participants said they often felt uncomfortable when giving doctors details of their medical history. They weren't familiar with medical language and were afraid they would forget important information. A smart card could be used anywhere, it could carry a lot of information and would reduce the possibility of misdiagnosis, mixing up notes and so on. German participants echoed these sentiments, arguing that it could also help to reduce costs by eliminating the need for repeat investigations. Polish participants liked the idea of a universal, comprehensive card that would be especially useful when travelling, in emergencies and accidents, and would be empowering for patients. People in Slovenia suggested that the patient's blood group and allergies could be printed visibly on the card so that these were immediately accessible in emergencies. Swiss participants felt the card would alleviate difficulties experienced by people who have a poor command of the local language, particularly relevant in a multilingual country like Switzerland. Participants in the UK thought the card would be useful for getting repeat prescriptions from the pharmacist, eliminating the need to make an appointment at the GP's surgery.

There were some concerns, however. Many people were worried about unauthorized access to the data on the card, especially since some of the information might be very sensitive. Participants in Poland and Switzerland felt that access should be restricted to doctors and emergency services and there should be safeguards to ensure that insurance companies and employers couldn't get hold of the information. Some British participants said they would be afraid of losing the card or forgetting to bring it when they had a doctor's appointment. They didn't want to be the sole carrier of their medical record, preferring the reassurance that someone else would share the responsibility.

Nevertheless, the overwhelming impression was of considerable enthusiasm for patient-held records. People are used to carrying credit cards in their bags or pockets. The risk of losing them or of breaches of security are outweighed by the advantages of convenience and freedom of movement. Medical smart cards appear to offer the same advantages.

Choosing where to receive care

The extent to which patients can exercise free choice of primary care doctor, specialist or hospital varies between the study countries. Choice is limited to a certain extent in every country. People who live in rural areas may have little choice because of travelling distances and restricted local facilities. Even in urban areas there are often administrative restrictions on where people can access health care, and in countries with GP gatekeeping systems, the choice of referral location is often made by the GP rather than the patient. Patients in Germany and Switzerland have the right to consult specialists directly, whereas patients in the other countries are expected to go via referral from their GP. In countries where health care is administered at county or regional level (e.g. Germany, Spain, Sweden and Switzerland) people are usually expected to receive treatment in local hospitals, although there is often some flexibility about this. On the other hand, people in countries such as Slovenia and Italy quite often travel outside their local area for elective hospital admissions.

The survey results provided evidence of a high demand for choice in each of the study countries, but people need information about the availability and quality of services to make informed choices and in most cases this is not available. With the exception of respondents in Spain and Switzerland, most people were dissatisfied with the opportunities for choice in their country. The majority felt they should be free to choose, but they were dissatisfied with the amount of information available to support these choices. However, not everyone saw choice as an unmitigated blessing. For example, participants in the Swedish focus groups expressed the view that patients should not have to worry about whether doctors have the necessary skills and they were not enthusiastic about having to invest time and effort in seeking out the best doctors. The survey confirmed the impression that Swedish people were much less enthusiastic about choice than those in the other countries.

Focus group participants were asked for their reactions to the publication of performance indicators which would allow public access to information on the quality of care among different health care providers. The response from many participants was enthusiastic. Participants in the Polish focus groups welcomed the idea of comprehensive national information disseminated through the mass media. They thought it would help them make choices and would act as a form of quality control, forcing the worst hospitals to improve. Italian participants wanted very detailed information about the safety, efficiency and technical quality of hospitals and specialist centres, and about the experience and reliability of doctors and other health professionals. Publication of performance indicators is already happening in the UK and is planned in Germany. People in Germany felt that publication of this type of information would help to encourage a more consumer-oriented approach among health care providers. British participants wanted more information about waiting times for particular specialties and specialists, success rates for specific operations and the qualifications of individual specialists.

There were some concerns, however. Some people in the UK felt there was a risk that publication of hospital league tables would increase the pressures on health professionals and staff might become demoralized if their hospital was not seen to be performing well. Meanwhile the 'best' hospitals might be swamped with patients and the quality of care might suffer as a result. They also pointed out that knowing where the best providers are is not much use if genuine choice doesn't exist. Some people felt that knowing more about performance variations would make people anxious by highlighting the weaknesses of the service rather than facilitating choice. Knowing that your local hospital is performing badly without being able to go elsewhere is unlikely to give patients a sense of empowerment. Indeed it could have quite the opposite effect. Participants in Germany and Poland were sceptical that health professionals would agree to publish the data openly. They felt performance information should be collected and published by an independent body to ensure its validity and trustworthiness.

In certain cases patients are free to go abroad for health care, particularly within the EU. All things being equal, most people prefer to receive their health care close to home, but there are signs that some, at least, are willing to contemplate the idea of travelling further afield. For example, many Germans, particularly younger people, indicated that they would be willing to travel elsewhere in Europe for health care. Swiss participants were more ambivalent about the idea. Switzerland is not a member of the EU, so opportunities to travel outside the country to obtain health care are limited, but some people go abroad for dental care or to purchase over-the-counter medicines or spectacles. On the one hand, encouraging people to 'shop around' in this way was seen as a good way of helping patients to take more responsibility, but on the other, there were concerns that it might lead to more 'medical tourism', driving costs up even further.

Our survey results demonstrate high levels of demand for more choice and greater patient autonomy among European patients. Attitudes to health care are becoming more consumerist and 'one size fits all' is no longer acceptable. Most people want to do as much as possible to help themselves when they are ill, but they also want flexible professional help which supports rather than undermines their efforts. Many are uncomfortable about placing themselves blindly in the hands of health professionals. Instead they want the assurance that they have selected the best person or the most appropriate treatment for their needs. They don't necessarily want to act independently (although the high demand for complementary therapies shows that an element of independent choice is popular), but they increasingly expect to be treated as partners by health professionals rather than as dependent victims of illness. Future generations of patients will be much less tolerant of medical paternalism.

PUBLIC INVOLVEMENT

Strengthening patients' rights

Legislation to protect patients' rights exists in each of the study countries. In recent years many governments have published patients' charters outlining these rights and there have been various campaigns to publicize them. Despite this, awareness of patients' rights appears low among both professionals and patients. Focus group participants tended to struggle when asked to list their rights, although in practice many knew quite a lot about what they were entitled to even if they didn't recognize this information as rights.

Many people said that patients' rights were frequently ignored and it was difficult for patients to claim their rights in the face of professional resistance. For example, in theory Swiss patients have the right to access their medical records and to have photocopies of them if they wish, but in practice medical records can be very difficult to obtain. Professionals were seen as closing ranks when criticized and patients felt powerless to challenge them. Patients' organizations usually focus on specific disease groups, often working in conjunction with health professionals to raise awareness of the needs of the people they represent, so they tend to be reluctant to criticize the medical profession. Consumer organizations that represent a broader constituency are sometimes more willing to hold a torch for patients' rights and to challenge professional authority if necessary. In several countries these groups have been at the forefront of efforts to raise the profile of patients' rights.

Participation in policy making

Encouraging greater public involvement in shaping health policy is beginning to be seen as a key plank of health care reform. For example, the UK government has taken steps to recruit lay people to serve on a wide range of committees and policy making bodies in the hope that they will encourage health professionals to take more account of the patient's perspective. In Germany, patients' organizations receive some statutory funding and are invited to participate in regional health conferences. In Poland, the government is providing support for self-help organizations and their representatives participate in various consultations. In Switzerland, the direct democratic system allows citizens to propose modifications to the law and the constitution, and there have been several attempts to modify the law on sickness insurance.

One might expect that these initiatives would be particularly necessary in countries, such as the UK, Poland or Slovenia, where health care is controlled and managed centrally. Local democratic control ought to be stronger and more responsive to local needs in countries where regional authorities administer the system and control the health care budget. Certainly the UK government seems to have gone further than most to correct the perceived democratic deficit in the health system. But in countries with more decentralized systems there is often a feeling that local politicians can't or won't represent patients' interests. For example, participants in the German focus groups felt members of self-help groups could do the job better. This may reflect wider alienation from the political process, or it may be a reaction to the greater power and influence of professional groups, but it strengthens the case for seeking new and better ways of securing public engagement in health policy making.

POLICY IMPLICATIONS

When looked at through the eyes of European patients it is clear that many health policy problems are shared. The similarities between our eight study countries were often more striking than the differences. People everywhere are concerned about waiting times, communication with health professionals, access to health information, continuity of care, involvement in decisions, flexibility and choice of providers and an equitable system for accessing health care resources according to need. They also want more autonomy and control over what happens to them and most people are keen to take more responsibility for managing their own health care.

There are no simple, structural solutions to these policy problems. None of the health systems is conspicuously better at meeting patients' needs than the others. There was no clear association between the method of funding, the extent of decentralization or the way in which access to care is organized and the responses and concerns of patients and the public. Politicians should be dissuaded from looking for 'big bang' solutions. There is much that is excellent about the way in which European health systems currently operate and the relatively high levels of public satisfaction are testimony to this. Since some countries are further down the road of reform than others, it can be instructive to examine the reactions of local people to various changes as they occur. There were many indications in our country studies of what patients want and several examples of good practice were described that could be built on and replicated elsewhere. We hesitate to make specific recommendations for fear of advocating the 'one size fits all' approach that we deplored earlier, but some possible policy responses are summarized briefly below.

Promoting partnerships with health professionals

No health system can function long without public support. This is why it is so important to learn from patients' experience and ensure that the system adapts to meet changing needs. Long waiting times are the most visible sign that all is not well as far as many patients are concerned. These problems require urgent solution, but few countries can afford to increase spending to the levels seen in

Switzerland and Germany, where capacity is greater and access appears much less problematic. Other, cheaper ways of solving the problem have to be found. Varying the skill mix by allowing people other than doctors to provide specific services would appear to offer considerable potential. Encouraging self-reliance and educating people to use health services appropriately may also prove effective. However, these initiatives will require fundamental changes in the way in which health care is delivered, in particular in the way health professionals relate to patients.

Health professionals, especially doctors, are held in very high regard by patients and members of the public, but attitudes and expectations are changing. People increasingly expect to be treated as partners in their care, but many medical staff still adopt paternalistic attitudes towards patients. Paternalism creates dependency, undermining people's self-confidence and ability to cope, so it is harmful to health and discordant with what the patient of the future will want.

Many doctors, nurses and other health professionals have not been trained to listen to patients and to take account of their preferences. They need better training in how to impart information, elicit patients' preferences and involve them in decision making. The best way to do this is to engage patients in the process of training health professionals. Direct feedback on patients' experiences can be very helpful and videos of consultations can be useful teaching aids. All health professionals should receive training in how to communicate with patients and skills should be monitored and updated as a key part of continuing professional development.

Communication skills training will help, but it won't be sufficient to create true partnerships between patients and professionals. What is needed is a fundamental change of attitude on both sides. Doctors and other health professionals must be prepared to share responsibility for decisions about clinical interventions. Shared decision making requires a commitment to offer choices, to share information, to clarify values and to share ownership of decisions made. Clinical care may have to be reorganized to allow more time for professional-patient discussion. Effective teamworking will be essential to achieving this goal. Professionals will need to ensure that patients understand the basis for their recommendations and must be willing to accept that patients' priorities and values may differ from theirs.

For their part, patients must accept responsibility for an enhanced role and must be prepared to ask questions and express their views. Patients' organizations should support patients in becoming critical consumers of health care. All medical interventions carry risk of harm as well as benefit and more is not always better. Careful selection of appropriate treatments is crucial to ensuring safety and treatment efficacy, and patients have an important role to play in this. Public education on how to assess risk and appraise medical advice could help to promote more cost-effective use of medical interventions.

Investing in information and advice

Our study provided clear evidence of the high demand for reliable, user-friendly health information. This includes the need for information about diseases and treatments and how to prevent illness and manage disease, but people also want information about the quality of care offered by different providers and support in making informed choices. At current rates of growth it seems likely that the majority of patients in most countries will be internet users within the next ten years or so. This will vastly increase the potential to meet these information needs. But access to reliable health information will not improve unless there is more public investment in good quality websites and information portals and more public education in critical appraisal of health information. Various initiatives have begun in our study countries and these should be strengthened and extended. There may be a case for a Europe-wide initiative to promote better access to reliable information. After all, the evidence base is universal and it would be relatively easy to translate and adapt materials that are developed in one country for use in another. It will also be important to provide free internet access in public places such as hospitals and clinics to minimize the risk of exacerbating the digital divide.

Access to health advice via a telephone helpline can be helpful. The British national patients' helpline, NHS Direct, may prove to be a model worth emulating but it is still too early to judge its impact on the system as a whole. Other examples of remote advice include email consultations and telemedicine. These need careful evaluation from the point of view of efficacy, safety and cost-effectiveness, but they may provide solutions to the widespread concerns about difficulties in getting quick access to health advice when it is needed.

Information and education to assist self-care is another area worthy of investment. This will be particularly relevant for patients with chronic diseases who need to become expert in managing their condition. Our study has revealed considerable demand for self-care among patients. People do not want to be entirely dependent on health professionals and prefer to be given tools for self-reliance whenever possible. A certain amount of self-management is essential for people with conditions such as diabetes, asthma, hypertension and so on. Time spent supporting them in this task can pay dividends in the longer term.

Support for continuity, flexibility and choice

Continuity of care is important to patients, but it doesn't necessarily have to mean always seeing the same doctor. Many patients are willing to see any one of a group of doctors in familiar surroundings if they know the doctors have access to reliable records giving them adequate knowledge of their medical history. People are also willing to consult other health professionals (e.g. nurses, therapists, pharmacists) if they are reassured that they have adequate training and experience to carry out the appropriate tasks. There is therefore considerable scope to vary skill mix and encourage teamworking, which in turn could improve speed of access.

The demand for continuity of care may appear to sit uneasily alongside the desire for more choice, but the two are not necessarily incompatible. The fact that people want to be able to choose their health care providers does not mean they want continual change. On the contrary, it seems very likely that people will remain loyal to providers they are happy with. What they seem to be expressing is a desire for a different relationship with public services, a sense that they have played an active part in selecting the people on whose advice and skill they will come to depend. People want to trust health providers, but trust is not the same as blind faith. Increasingly patients are looking for evidence that the health care providers who are advising and treating them are doing the best job possible. This is an inevitable consequence of better education, less deference and growing confidence in their dealings with professionals. As such it should be welcomed, but it requires reciprocal action on the part of providers. It means they will have to be willing to subject themselves to external monitoring and public disclosure of the results. Defensive reactions will only make matters worse, undermining trust and fostering suspicion.

If choice is to become a practical reality it will require sufficient capacity among providers to cater for different needs, publication of quality indicators to support informed choices and to encourage greater responsiveness, and relaxation of bureaucratic restrictions to allow patients greater freedom. The popularity of the electronic patient-held record or smart card among our study participants was interesting because it can be seen as a passport to empowerment and greater choice. If you can carry your medical record around with you, you control access to it and the card enables you to consult a range of providers without having to worry that you may forget crucial details of your medical history. As long as people are reassured that there are robust data protection systems in place to ensure confidentiality of personal information, patient-held records have the potential to transform relationships. Patients have a right to know what is being communicated about them between professionals and they should be encouraged to read their medical notes. Records could be stored on secure websites, with access controlled by patients themselves via smart cards. This way the patient, not the doctor, becomes the rightful 'owner' of the record.

Maintaining trust in health systems

Policy makers everywhere struggle with the need to control health care costs while satisfying raised public expectations. By encouraging patients and citizens to play a more active role in health care and health improvement, they hope to promote appropriate use of cost-effective services. The extent to which this is recognized and acted upon as a key plank of health system reform varies between our study countries. Initiatives to strengthen patients' rights, to provide financial and other support for patients' organizations and to involve their representatives in policy making bodies are common to many countries and are undoubtedly useful. But there is much more that could be done.

Most people are not members of organized patients' groups and only a minority want to sit on policy committees or seek legal redress to secure their rights. What most people want is the security of knowing that health services will be there when they need them, that their views and preferences will be taken account of by health professionals, that they will be given the help they need to help themselves, that they can access all the information they need to know about their condition and the treatment options, and that they won't have to worry about the financial consequences of being ill. European patients also want to be sure that these benefits are equitably distributed and that public resources are being used efficiently for the good of all. Social solidarity is the essential underpinning of a sustainable health system.

Public involvement in, and democratic accountability for, decisions about health care priorities, including decisions about what is affordable out of public resources, will become more and more essential. Public ignorance of the issues breeds unrealistic aspirations and inappropriately simplistic political responses. Transparent procedures are crucial at both national and local levels and should be embedded into the governance of health systems. People value their health services and want to feel ownership of them. Policy makers should do all they can to encourage this sense of engagement.

Ultimately effective public engagement depends on the prior establishment of more equal partnerships between patients and health professionals. If people are treated like passive dependents when they seek health care, it is unlikely that they will be able to play their full part as active citizens, helping to shape health policy decisions. Attempts to create a complex superstructure of public consultation and involvement will founder if the basic building blocks are not firmly embedded. The really important changes need to occur at the level of individual interactions between patients and health professionals. The development of a more active role for patients will be fundamental to securing the future of European health systems.

APPENDIX a
LITERATURE REVIEW
TEMPLATE

1 Aims

To review available literature on patients' attitudes to likely future developments in health and health care.

To highlight gaps in knowledge and issues which require further exploration in focus groups and/or surveys.

2 Methods

A brief (about 10,000 words), critical and selective review of published and 'grey' literature which examines and collates data on existing patterns of access to information and care, and attitudes to the patient's role, paying special attention to differences between age groups, gender, socioeconomic status and ethnic group where relevant.

To facilitate comparison between countries, it is important that the review covers each of the topics listed below, even if there is little relevant information available. If nothing is known about a particular topic, the review should make this clear. The review should draw on good quality empirical data wherever possible. Unsubstantiated commentaries should not be included unless they are particularly interesting or important.

An advisory group should be established in each country to guide the work of the reviewer. Membership should include a local representative of MSD and, in Germany, Sweden and Switzerland only, the manager of the local office of the Picker Institute. Other members could include health professionals and policy makers, patients' representatives and academics. Groups could meet on one or two occasions to advise on sources of information and to comment on the draft review.

3 Sources

- Published literature on health policy
- Major medical and nursing journals
- Government publications
- Reports of patient organizations and consumer groups
- Internet
- Newspapers

Literature search restricted to articles published since 1990 within each country.

4 Topics to be included

a) General attitudes to the health care system:

- Public support for/criticisms of current system
- Views on payment systems
- Patients' rights and responsibilities
- Perceptions of likely future changes in health care
- Political debates about health policy
- Public involvement in health policy making

b) Quality of health care:

- General attitudes to quality of health care. How do patients evaluate quality of care?
- Medical errors and patient safety
- Access and waiting times, including emergency and out-of-hours care, and telephone advice
- Relationships with health professionals, including communication skills
- Trust in health professionals
- Continuity of care
- Paternalism versus patient empowerment/patient-centred care
- Opportunities for involvement in decisions about treatment – shared decision making

c) Health and health care information:

- Extent of demand for health information – do people want it? Can they get what they want/need?
- Current and preferred sources of advice on health problems, treatments, availability and quality of health services
- Access to medical records
- Confidentiality/data protection
- Use of internet to access health information – Who uses it now? Who will use it in the future?

d) Consumerism in health care

- Views on equity/inequalities in access
- Attitudes to individual versus public good
- Limits on demand (e.g. cost-containment strategies)
- Health care as a consumer good?
- Limits to consumerism?
- Attitudes to priority-setting and rationing

e) Where health care is delivered

- Patients' attitudes to, and preferences for, primary, secondary and tertiary care, care in the home
- Willingness to travel within country to receive care
- Willingness to travel across country borders to receive care
- Likely impact of future changes, including telemedicine and remote diagnostics

f) Who delivers health care?

- Patients' perceptions of doctors, nurses and pharmacists
- Self-diagnosis, self-medication, self-care, including 'over-the-counter' medicines, self-help groups
- Use of alternative and complementary therapies for self-medication and use recommended by physicians

g) Future developments in screening and treatment

- Attitudes to, and availability of, new or innovative medicines
- Attitudes to, and availability of, genetic testing

- Attitudes to, and availability of, 'lifestyle medicines' (e.g. hair loss treatments) at personal cost versus state cost
- Co-payment for tests or treatment
- Do patients feel they have a choice of treatment? Do they want more choice?

APPENDIX b
FOCUS GROUP TOPIC GUIDE

Welcome from facilitator (5 mins)

Introductions (5 mins)

Each participant to introduce him or herself – say their name, bit about their family background, what they do for a living

Warm up (15 mins)

Discuss patients' own experience – last time they went to see a clinician? How often? Who do they see?

What do you think of health care in this country? Good things, bad things? Will it be there for you in the future?

What changes have you noticed in the past five years?

What changes do you think might happen in the future? *Probe specifically: do they expect to pay more in the future?* How positive or negative are you about these changes?

What would you like to see changing?

Quality

In some of the focus groups, as a way of getting people to think about their experiences of the health service in more detail and what they would like to be different in the future, a discussion was structured around what constitutes a 'good' quality experience of the health service.

What things do you think are most important when you're thinking about creating a 'good quality' health service?

Probe: having choice, easy access, quick access, being treated with respect, having time to talk through your symptoms and understand what you're being told, seeing the same person throughout your treatment rather than lots of different people, seeing a doctor or specialist face-to-face, knowing how to complain if you have a problem, being able to ask further questions if you need to, being provided with lots of information, knowing your doctor well, having information about the medicines you are taking, having information about new therapies; having a choice of therapies, having access to new therapies.

Note: The list above may be presented on a handout with respondents asked to tick the most important and least important things for them.

What else is important?

Trade-offs: What changes are good? And which are bad for patients? (25 mins)

The way that health services are delivered in the future is likely to change. We're going to look at some of the ways in which this might happen and find out which changes you think are worth making and which you think, as a patient, you would not like. Try not to get stuck in how things work now and think about how health care might work in the future.

HANDOUT 1: future scenarios (see end of document)

For each:

What do you like about this idea? What don't you like?

What would be the benefits for patients?

Overall, which of these changes do you feel would be most significant? Which are you more concerned about?

Moderator to explain that for the rest of the discussion we are going to focus on three different areas of health care in the future (for the groups lasting an hour and three quarters it may be that we only have time to get through two of the issues):

(1) How can the information revolution play a part?
(2) What role can the patient play?
(3) Who will run services?

**Issue 1: How can the information revolution play a part?
(15–20 mins)**

What sources of information do you currently use?

Probe: leaflets, internet, TV, magazines, newspapers, friends etc.

When do you seek out information? When do you rely on others providing it?
What information is it important for patients to know?

Probe: details of condition, treatment, treatment options, information about doctors/specialists, past performance of hospital, information about medicines

When you do seek out information, are you satisfied with what you find? Do you find answers to the questions most important to you?
How confident are you about acting on advice that you read? In what situations would you be likely to do this? When would it be inappropriate? When would you want to follow it up by seeing someone?
What questions do you ask when you see a doctor/nurse/specialist?

Probe: do they tend to hold back or are they comfortable asking questions?

If you were advising someone else who was going to see a doctor or perhaps was due to have an operation, what advice would you give them for when they're talking to health professionals? What questions would you advise them to ask?
Card sort – list of sources of information presented on different cards for individual to sort: family and friends, internet, magazines, newspapers, TV programmes, GP, pharmacist, nurses, community health visitors, specialists, medicine companies, patient groups, telephone helplines

Get group to sort the cards in different ways:

Which of these sources of information do you trust most?
Which do you trust least?
Which of these sources of information do you find most accessible/easy to use?
And which are less so?

Internet/email
Would you feel happy using the Internet to find out about . . .?

Probe: medicines, services and tests, doctor's performance, advice about leading a healthy lifestyle, a second opinion, an email consultation?

What would make you more confident?

Issue 2: What role will the patient play? Rights and responsibilities (15–20 mins)

What things do you take control of at the moment in terms of your own health care? When you're ill at the moment, what do you do? What do you feel happy doing on your own?

Probe: monitor own medicines, take supplements not prescribed by GP, exercise, go for regular check-ups, eat healthily, buy over-the-counter medicines

What things do you think are your responsibility? And what things do you think are the responsibility of others (e.g. your GP or hospital specialist)?

Probe: how dependent on health professionals are they?

How would you feel about taking on more responsibility as an individual?

Probe: tests for particular diseases, monitoring your blood pressure at home, doing more exercise, eating more healthily, going to the pharmacist first

How would you feel about taking on more responsibility as more sophisticated self-diagnosis and genetic tests are developed for conditions such as cancer and heart disease?

Probe: would you be likely to use such a test? What sort of things for? What if you knew there was no cure for the condition?

Do you feel you are given enough information about the different choices and options available to you? *e.g. if there are treatment options in addition to what is being recommended*

Do you feel in control when you are a patient?

Probe: is there a difference if you pay for your own treatment?

Are there times when you would like to have more of a say/more control? If so, when?

Typically, how well do you adhere to your doctor's advice or treatment? Do you feel that it would be easier to adhere to your treatment regimen if you had more information about the condition? And about the recommended treatment?

What rights do feel you have as a patient?

Probe: choice, complaints, privacy and confidentiality

Are there further rights that you think you should have?

Probe: right to access different treatment options, right to a second opinion, right to be spoken to by someone who speaks your own language, right to be treated with dignity, right to treatment for 'life-style' indications – e.g. should state pay for treatments for baldness, non-clinical obesity, impotence?

Issue 3: Who will run services? (15–20 mins)

Who do you currently come into contact with when talking about health?

Probe: doctors, nurses, community visitors, patients' groups, charities/ voluntary groups, pharmacists, surgeons, specialists, friends and family, alternative medicine practitioners etc.?

What are your perceptions of each of the different health professionals?

Probe: who are they most likely to ask questions of? Who do they have easiest access to? Who understands their needs best? Who do they trust most?

Nurses
How would you feel if nurses took on more of a role?

What if your local doctors' surgery were run primarily by nurses rather than doctors?

How confident would you feel in nurses prescribing medicines?

Pharmacists

What do you think about pharmacists taking on a greater role in providing health services – for example being able to prescribe more medicines over the counter?

What sort of medicines?

What, if anything, would need to be different at your local pharmacist to make you feel more confident?

How would you feel about complementary medicine and therapies becoming more mainstream? Would you have as much trust in complementary practitioners? Have you used them before? Did you tell your doctor/ was your doctor involved? Can you imagine using them in the future?

Thanks and conclusion (10 mins)

Which idea do you think might have most impact – for the better – for patients?

And which are you most concerned about?

In the future

...everyone could carry around their medical history on a smart card – a type of electronic card that stores lots of individual data. This would mean that it would be easier to move around and see different doctors and you wouldn't have to keep telling people the same information.

...patients may be able to access much more information about the performance of doctors, specialists and hospitals all over the country – from the quality of care given in the past experience of a doctor. Patients may then choose where to go for treatment based on this information. They may travel further afield to be seen by a particular specialist or because they will be seen more quickly. Or they might choose to wait longer to be seen by the person who they think is best for the job.

...patients may be diagnosed and treated with the aid of telemedicine. This would mean that you could talk to medical specialists using a live telephone and video link – this could be from your local surgery or even from your own home. It would mean that you wouldn't have the consultation in person, however.

...the telephone might be used much more as a way of accessing information and advice as a patient. You wouldn't see the doctor or nurse in person but you would be able to access the advice when you needed it, quickly and around the clock. It might also mean that you could have a consultation with a top specialist from another part of the country or even another part of the world.

...rather than always seeing the same doctor you might make an appointment to see one of a range of doctors who are available. You would be able to get an appointment more quickly but you wouldn't see the same doctor every time.

APPENDIX c
TELEPHONE SURVEY
QUESTIONNAIRE

We are interested to learn more about people's views on choice in the health care system, including choice of provider, choice of physician and choice of treatment.

1   Have you received any health care in the last 12 months?
    (include visits to local doctors and other health care providers for any reason)

    - Yes I visited a doctor
    - I didn't visit a doctor, but I visited a nurse or other health care provider
    - No → go to 9

2   When was your last (most recent) visit to a health facility or provider? Was it

    - In the last 30 days?
    - 1–3 months ago?
    - More than 3 but less than 6 months ago?
    - Between 6 and 12 months ago?
    - Don't remember

3   In the last 12 months, how often did the doctor(s) (nurses or other health care providers) listen carefully to you?

    - Always
    - Usually
    - Sometimes
    - Never

4   In the last 12 months, how often did the doctor(s) (nurses or

other health care providers) explain things in a way you could understand?

- Always
- Usually
- Sometimes
- Never

5 In the last 12 months, how often did the doctor(s) (nurses or other health care providers) give you time to ask questions about your health problem or treatment?

- Always
- Usually
- Sometimes
- Never

6 In the last 12 months, when you went for health care, were any decisions made about your care, treatment (giving you medicines, for example), or tests?

- Yes
- No → go to 9

7 In the last 12 months, how often did the doctor(s) (nurses or other health care providers) involve you as much as you wanted to be in deciding about your care, treatment or tests?

- Always
- Usually
- Sometimes
- Never

8 Now, overall how would you rate your experience of how well health care providers communicated with you in the last 12 months?

- Very good
- Good
- Moderate
- Bad
- Very bad

9 In general, when you need medical treatment and more than one treatment is available, who do you think should make the decision about which treatment is best for you?

- I should decide
- I should make the decision after consulting my doctor
- My doctor and I should decide together
- My doctor should make the decision after discussion with me
- My doctor should decide

10 Do you feel you have sufficient information about new treatments to choose the best one for you?

- Yes → go to question 12
- No → go to question 11
- Don't know → go to question 11
- Not applicable → go to question 11

11 If no or don't know, what do you find dissatisfying about the information available to you?

- I have not been able to find any information
- The information available is confusing, hard to understand
- I don't trust the information available
- The information available is conflicting
- Other (please specify)

12 Where or from whom would you normally expect to find information about new treatments?

- General practitioner
- Medical specialist
- Friends/family
- Public library
- Television programmes
- Newspapers or magazines
- Internet
- Advertisements
- Pharmacist
- Patient group
- Other (please specify)

13 In general, if you need to consult a primary care doctor do you think you should have a free choice about which doctor to consult?

- Yes
- No
- Don't know

14 Do you feel you have sufficient information about primary care doctors to choose the best one for you?

- Yes
- No
- There is no choice
- Don't want to choose
- Don't know

15 In general, if you need to consult a specialist doctor do you think you should have a free choice about which doctor to consult?

- Yes
- No
- Don't know

16 Do you feel you have sufficient information about specialist doctors to choose the best one for you?

- Yes
- No
- There is no choice
- Don't want to choose
- Don't know

17 In general, if you need to go to hospital do you think you should have a free choice of which hospital to go to?

- Yes
- No
- Don't know

18 Do you feel you have sufficient information about hospitals to choose the best one for you?

- Yes
- No
- There is no choice
- Don't want to choose
- Don't know

19 Now, overall how would you rate the opportunities for patients in this country to make choices about their health care?

- Very good
- Good

- Moderate
- Bad
- Very bad
- Don't know

20 What is the highest level of formal education you have completed to date?

- No education
- Primary education
- Secondary education (high school)
- University degree

INDEX

THE GLOBAL CHALLENGE OF HEALTH CARE RATIONING

Angela Coulter and Chris Ham (eds)

Rationing or priority setting occurs in all health care systems. Doctors, managers and politicians are involved in making decisions on how to use scarce resources and which groups and patients should receive priority. These decisions may be informed by the results of medical research and cost effectiveness studies but they also involve the use of judgement and experience. Consequently, priority setting involves ethics as well as economics and decisions on who should live and who should die remain controversial and contested.

This book seeks to illuminate the debate on priority setting by drawing on experience from around the world. The authors are all involved in priority setting, either as decision makers or researchers, and their contributions demonstrate in practical terms how different countries and disciplines are approaching the allocation of resources between competing claims. Accessible to general readers a well as specialists, *The Global Challenge of Health Care Rationing* summarizes the latest thinking in this area and provides a unique resource for those searching for a guide through the maze.

Contents

c. 228 pp   0 335 20463 5 (Paperback)   0 335 20464 3 (Hardback)

REGULATING HEALTHCARE
A PRESCRIPTION FOR IMPROVEMENT?

Kieran Walshe

Healthcare organizations in the UK and the USA face a growing tide of regulation, accreditation, inspection and external review, aimed at improving their performance. In the USA, over three decades of healthcare regulation by state and federal government and by non-governmental agencies have created a complex, costly and overlapping network of oversight arrangements for healthcare organizations. In the UK's government run National Health Service, regulation is central to current health policy, with the creation of a host of new national agencies and inspectorates tasked with overseeing the performance of NHS hospitals and other organizations.

But does regulation work? This book:

- explores the development and use of healthcare regulation in both countries, comparing and contrasting their experience and drawing on regulatory research in other industries and settings
- offers a structured approach to analysing what regulators do and how they work
- develops principles for effective regulation, aimed at maximizing the benefits of regulatory interventions and minimizing their costs

Regulating Healthcare will be read by those with an interest or involvement in health policy and management, including policy makers, healthcare managers, health professionals and students. It is particularly suitable for use on postgraduate health and health related programmes.

Contents

c. 224 pp   0 335 21022 8 (Paperback)   0 335 21023 6 (Hardback)